Making Sense of Organizati Change and Innovation in Health Care

This book explores the hospital as a health care organization via everyday ethnography, an approach that involves a mix of fieldwork methods designed to analyze the everyday change process which includes participatory observation, qualitative interviews, and shadowing.

One way to define a hospital is by its high level of formal organization, resulting in written or digital communication as the main source of communication in patient journals, minutes, and medical and quality guidelines. In contrast, in this book, the aspects of the informal organization will be the focus. In spite of the many formal regulations of health care, hospitals are also chaotic organizing places where many different groups of people interact in order to negotiate, to practice, and to make sense of daily work tasks. The underlying argument is that, in the mundane everyday life of hospitals, frontline workers and their interactions with patients and local managers remain at the core of organizing hospitals. The overall purpose of this book is to report back from the field of health care, demonstrating how people, their interactions and narratives become important elements of organizing hospitals.

The book will be of interest to students and scholars in and across health care management, organization studies, ethnography, sociology, qualitative methods, anthropology, service management, and cultural studies.

Anne Reff Pedersen is a professor with special responsibilities in public organization and innovation at the Department of Organization at Copenhagen Business School, Denmark.

Routledge Studies in Health Management

Edited by Ewan Ferlie

The health care sector is now of major significance, economically, scientifically and societally. In many countries, health care organizations are experiencing major pressures to change and restructure, while cost containment efforts have been accentuated by global economic crisis. Users are demanding higher service quality, and health care professions are experiencing significant reorganization whilst operating under increased demands from an ageing population.

Critically analytic, politically informed, discursive and theoretically grounded, rather than narrowly technical or positivistic, the series seeks to analyse current health care organizations. Reflecting the intense focus of policy and academic interest, it moves beyond the day to day debate to consider the broader implications of international organizational and management research and different theoretical framings.

Making Sense of Organizational Change and Innovation in Health Care

An Everyday Ethnography

Anne Reff Pedersen

Routledge
Taylor & Francis Group

LONDON AND NEW YORK

First published 2020 by Routledge

2 Park Square, Milton Park, Abingdon, Oxon, OX14 4RN
605 Third Avenue, New York, NY 10017

Routledge is an imprint of the Taylor & Francis Group, an informa business

First issued in paperback 2020

Library of Congress Cataloging-in-Publication Data
A catalog record for this title has been requested

ISBN: 978-0-367-14062-5 (hbk)
ISBN: 978-0-367-77692-3 (pbk)

Typeset in Sabon
by Apex CoVantage, LLC

Contents

Acknowledgments

This book is the product of a ten-year study of processes of organizational change and innovation in health care organizations. Many people have helped me along the way: researchers, practitioners, public managers, and patients. I am indebted to all of them. First of all, this book was not possible without the openness and invitations from public health care organizations. I would like to thank all the members of the research group of POVI (Public Organization, Value and Innovation) and all the former members of CHM (Center of Health Management) at CBS, in particular Mette Brehm Johansen, Susanne Boch Waldorff, Carsten Greve, Mie Plotnikof, and Vibeke Kristine Scheller. Karina Sehested, Eva Sørensen, and Ewan Ferlie have also been helpful colleagues. Thanks.

1 Introduction

Making Sense of Organizational Change and Innovation
in Health Care: An Everyday Ethnography

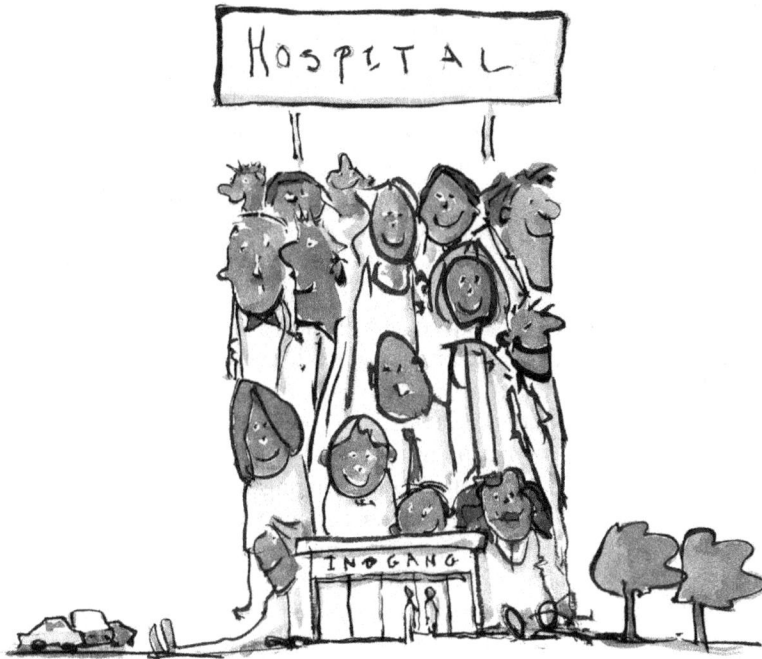

Source: Ahlefeldt-Laurvig

Encountering Everyday Life Through Meeting People

Many books and articles have been published on health care organizations in the last two decades or more. From a sociological and organizational perspective, studies have explored social and institutional systems (Goffman, 1968), the birth of the clinic (Foucault, 1973), the power of medicine (Turner, 1983), medical practice (Mol, 2002), institutional change (Scott, Ruef, Mendel, & Caronna, 2000), and organizing (Ferlie, 2016). One could then ask, "Do we really need more books about this topic?" After reading Finn Borum's (1995) 1976 field study, I was incredulous that, even 40 years on, some of the same conflicts are still present in hospitals today. For instance, the large degree of autonomy surgical wards have when planning/cancelling operations, how doctor conferences are performed, and how clinical wards obtain status regarding their number of beds. Many of these issues are still relevant today because everyday routines such as bathing (Goffman, 1968), medical conferences, and operations (Borum, 1995) are still daily activities at hospital wards, confirming that everyday life in health care organizations are dominated by strongly routine, negotiated practices. After more than 15 years of conducting field studies at hospitals, I returned to a clinical ward that I had studied many years ago. The hospital had undergone change several times by adopting various management models and the ward had become a functional unit/department that was now part of a center. I asked the nurses and doctors on the ward about what had changed since my last visit. They responded, "Nothing, down here, we see patients just like we always have." This empirical account supports the notion that change is perceived as a difficult process in hospitals, and even if management models and concepts continually change, everyday clinical life has its own time, pace, and way of doing things (Pedersen, 2009).

Still, recent societal trends have led to changes in hospital conditions: patient stays are shorter, IT facilities are making e-consulting more appealing, and politicians are demanding improved productivity, budget cuts, and faster patient trajectories (Nickelsen, 2019). So, worldwide changes in society are reflected by modifications in health care organizations, which are not isolated islands but part of a more global, digitalized, and individualized society (Ferlie, Montgomery, & Pedersen, 2016). As a result, contemporary studies of everyday life in health care organizations are always relevant, as they reflect our changing society while simultaneously mirroring the battle between dominant values and routines and new societal demands. These battles do not always end in bloody wars but are often dealt with in the everyday negotiations of employees and patients. The mundane, everyday practices of local employees and their collaboration with external stakeholders are at the core of any health care community; thus, their narratives are the focus of this book.

This book explores everyday life in health care organizations using organizational ethnography, an approach that involves a mixture of fieldwork methods (Hammersley & Atkinson, 2007; Neyland, 2007) designed to analyze organizations, e.g., the hospital, which includes participatory observation, qualitative interviews, shadowing, and document studies (Pope, 2005). Organizational ethnography applies not only to certain methods used to describe organizations but also to theorizing and understanding organizations using specific kinds of data. This means that, from an organizational ethnography perspective, health care organizations are defined by social interactions, relationships, and social dynamics, all of which represent activities that can be observed, talked about, and interpreted (Pedersen & Humle, 2016). When using an organizational ethnography perspective, it is not possible to present a complete picture of change processes in health care organizations, which is why this book employs a bricolage of snapshots of the narratives people tell in their everyday work life to show how sensemaking and value negotiations consistently play central roles in organizational change processes.

> *The purpose of this book is to explore how people in health care organizations use narratives to make sense of different organizational change processes in their everyday work life.*

Health care organizations are meeting places for people, and their narratives and sensemaking of organizational change processes in everyday life become the focus of analysis. As the purpose of this book is to investigate everyday contexts, local employees are, thus, considered central to studying and understanding the surrounding narratives of change processes. New research on materiality, nonhuman actors, and digitalization has gained recent attention in science and technology studies of health care, addressing new and emerging conditions for organizing (Allen, 2002). Both in line and in contrast to many of these detailed science and technology studies, this book addresses the human aspects of a health care organization by acknowledging how people and their interactions and sensemaking continue to play central roles in changing health care organizations.

One way to describe everyday life in health care organization is by its high level of formal organization, resulting in digital communication by patient journals, medical guidelines, and quality standards as the main source of organizing. This book focuses on another way to describe everyday life through the informal organizing, as in spite of the many formal regulations, health care organizations are also chaotic meeting places, where health care professionals are negotiating to make sense of their everyday work tasks. The underlying argument in this book is that, despite new technologies and complex contemporary health care issues, the mundane, everyday lives of organizational members, and their interactions with external relations as patients (McDermott & Pedersen, 2016), remain a core element of organizational change in health care organizations. Even though we have read about these relationships before, contemporary narratives of the frontline workers remain a never-ending field of exploration for providing vital insights into organizational change processes in health care.

Organizational Change as Ongoing Sensemaking in Everyday Organizing

Health care organizations reflect the societies that surround them; a current pressure in Western society is to deliver faster patient trajectories and to innovate more efficient treatments plans to meet the individualized patient needs and the societal needs of a growing chronic and elderly patient population (Ferlie et al., 2016). Therefore, in one health care vision, health care organizations are fast-moving organizations, becoming the meeting place for new technological and digital development and expanding the possibilities of medicine and for contemporary social and economic population health issues, such as health equality, lifestyle consequences, and longer life expectancy. In another vision, health care organizations remain the same; they are populated by health professionals with strong health care values, having formalized routines and evidence-based work tasks, with strict validation, guidelines, and assessment practices. Thereby, health care organizations can both be viewed as places of resistance toward change and as places with accelerated change processes (Ferlie et al., 2005).

In the organization theory literature, organizational change is divided into studies of episodic change and continuous change, where the former understands organizations as stable entities and the latter understands organizations as an ongoing movement (Weick & Quinn, 1999). This book defines organizational change from a continuous change perspective, which means that change processes are part of the ongoing organizing process. A sensemaking organizing change perspective relates to how participants in organizational change understand and make sense of change processes; thus a sensemaking perspective on organizational change has the ability to provide essential meaning for maintaining or reproducing stability and/or promoting resistance to change in and around organizations (Vaara, Sonenshein, & Boje, 2016). A sensemaking perspective on organizational change provides valuable insight into how participants make sense of change projects and processes and how they support or resist change processes. These organizational change processes are also related to local values and multiple logics (Reay & Hinings, 2009).

The change projects presented in this book were all identified through organizational ethnography. This means that the empirically presented change projects in the chapters are not the results of an overall theoretical change framework or a certain way of understanding elements of organizational change. Thus, these change projects were identified through a bottom-up approach asking about current change projects in the health care organizations. Different field studies will have found other projects. Together, these local change projects are examples that illustrate the everyday human organizing perspective because they are unpredictable change projects and themes, maybe even mundane change examples, but nevertheless current and thereby relevant change processes for the participants involved. They include a large group of different people: patients, health care professionals, clinical managers, and external stakeholders, such as innovation consultants, administrators, regional politicians, and state policymakers because local change projects are often not intra-organizational processes. Instead, local change projects become part of everyday organizing as ongoing organizing processes of the past, present, and future (Hernes, 2014), which means that they require sensemaking, negotiations, and narratives because they often result in unintended organizing consequences. When talking with people about organizational change, a sensemaking and narrative perspective is the inevitable approach.

A Pragmatic Narrative Framework

A very simple argument about organizational change and its relation to sensemaking is that if people do not understand the meaning of a given problem or change idea, they will likely resist it. People need meaning to interact and function (Bruner, 1991; Gabriel, 2000), which is also the case for the people working and entering organizations as they make sense out of organizing in an effort to understand, legitimize, and act. In that way, organizing is intertwined with narratives (Czarniawska, 1997). Sometimes narratives are told as individual narratives, by one storyteller, e.g., a clinical manager or a patient. Other times, narratives are told as the shared narratives of many storytellers, sharing a sense of the same events, e.g., from a group of health care professionals. The following chapters present an analysis of individual and shared narratives.

The narrative approach presented in this book is a pragmatic narrative understanding that includes different types of narratives. This means that the narrative framework includes more than one definition of a narrative because organizational narratives reflect their complex and dynamic surroundings and therefore come in many forms. Some organizational narratives are fragmented, often defined as ante- (pre-) narratives, with a fragmented structure and no coherence of plots or events but often told as contradictory narratives with tensions, ambiguity, and discontinuity, and therefore drawing on diverse and fragmented storytelling (Boje, 2001; Cunliffe, Luhman, & Boje, 2004; Pedersen & Humle, 2016; Vaara et al., 2016). Other organizational narratives are structured where a chain of events directs a plot or causal relationships between the events. These narratives are often told to persuade others to follow an idea and can be defined as strategic spokesperson narratives (Gabriel, 2000; Akrich, Callon, Latour, & Monaghan, 2002; Pedersen & Johansen, 2012). Some studies have combined these narratives, arguing that both structured and more provisory narratives are useful in studies of organizing, change, and innovation processes because they both have the capacity to direct and make sense of coordination (Bartel & Garud, 2009). In the following chapters, both fragmented and structured narratives will be presented in more detail. An empirical insight from the chapters is that fragmented narratives are often found in individual narratives and structured narratives are mostly found in the shared narratives of many storytellers. Both individual and shared narratives can be presented as fragmented or structured narratives, as narrative theory has no explanation for their different forms, only that they are told in different situated surroundings that reflect their structure (Boje, 2001).

Common to both fragmented and more structured narratives is that they all entail storytellers telling their personal stories, i.e., they are the characters who act in the stories, with different intentions and events that are linked to the characters. Consequently, the telling of characters and events is the building block of narratives. Thus the main contribution of using a narrative perspective in studies of organizational change processes is to show how organizing does not happen because of only shared narratives, values, or dominant logics. Instead, the analyses demonstrate how a central condition of making sense of change processes is that this happens through multiple narratives. Some of these narratives never meet, others relate, but together they create opportunities for organizing change in and around hospitals.

The research questions are:

> *How can we understand organizational change by doing an everyday ethnography?*

> *Which narratives can be found when making sense of organizational change processes?*

> *In addition, what are the sensemaking consequences for organizational change processes?*

These research questions are addressed by illustrating different narratives from four field studies and demonstrating how theses narratives make sense of situated everyday change processes. First, Chapter 2 is theoretical, unfolding a narrative framework in relation to understanding organizational change. Chapters 3 through 7 are analytical, illustrating a collage of different narratives and sensemaking conditions for organizational change processes in an everyday context. The analytical chapters are not presented in chronological order but in a funnel optic, starting with a presentation of individual narratives at a ward and concluding with national and policy narratives. This approach presents organizational change processes in an everyday context from the individual to macro-levels, illustrating that narratives of organizational change relate to other narratives and never take place in isolation.

Everyday Ethnographical Studies

A short description of each of the four everyday ethnographic studies will now be presented. Ybema, Yanow, Wels, and Kamsteeg (2009) defined several aspects of everyday life studies using organizational ethnography. They noted that a combination of methods and a description of the work scene draw close to explicit and often overlooked tacit knowledge and are context-sensitive (p. 9). All four studies combine different types of methods, ranging from interviews, observation, and participation in workshops, to document studies and shadowing, so they describe organizational change processes from an everyday perspective, from the hospital ward or from the daily meeting activities. They collect narratives from the field, and what can be described as backstage narratives, from the work scenes, as they entail everyday events. The interviews were conducted in meeting rooms, in hallways, or in employees' offices as part of doing the field studies. Many of the studies were also part of larger research collaborations, which means they were not done by a single researcher but by collaborations in communities of researchers.

Study 1: The Introduction of a New Triage Model in an Emergency Ward

This ethnographic study followed the implementation of a new triage visitation process for prioritizing incoming patients at the emergency ward at a regional hospital. The patients arrived by ambulance, were referred by their general practitioner, or came in on their own initiative. The emergency ward consisted of an emergency unit and an observation unit where patients were sent after having been assessed and the treatment initiated. From the observation unit, patients were either discharged or referred to specialized wards in the hospital. The implementation of the new triage model involved work standardization and coding the incoming patients with colors (green, yellow, orange, or red) to reflect the urgency of their need for assessment. The change process involved nurses, doctors, and managers at the emergency ward, as well as patients, indirectly, as they did not know about the color codes but were waiting at the emergency ward to receive hospital services.

Methods: Both semi-structured, qualitative interviews and participatory observations were conducted as part of the fieldwork. The observations were carried out as place-based and person-based observations— so-called shadowing (Czarniawska-Joerges, 2007). The observations included a participatory element consisting mainly of questioning and reasoning together with the nurses in their triage work and while performing simple, practical tasks in relation to general nursing in the ward. Most of the observations took place during daytime hours in the emergency ward, although observations were also conducted to a lesser extent during evening and night shifts. In this case, the researcher followed employees in their daily work, focusing particularly on triage-related activities. In total, 21 semi-structured individual interviews were conducted, primarily with nurses but also with doctors, managers, and patients in the emergency ward. All interviews were conducted using thematically arranged interview guides, in which the topics and issues to be covered were specified, though room was left to allow other relevant topics to surface and be explored during the interview. Each interview lasted 40–80 minutes and took place in the emergency ward. Interviews were recorded and subsequently transcribed for thematic coding and analysis. The data material used is based on both interviews and observation notes.[1]

Study 2: Changing the Nurse Education and Everyday Organizing in a Rehabilitation Ward

This ethnographic study followed the everyday life in a ward of a rehabilitation hospital. The rehabilitation hospital is responsible for the rehabilitation of patients after treatment in orthopedic, rheumatologic, medical, and neurological wards in other hospitals. The patients are often amputees, arthritis patients, and those coping with cerebral hemorrhages or injuries sustained in a fall. The health care professionals were nurses, physicians, assistant nurses, a social counselor, and a large number of occupational therapists and physiotherapists. At the clinic, nurses and doctors work side by side with the patients. The therapists and social counselors have separate locations at the hospitals, so the patients go to therapist training sessions from the clinic. While conducting fieldwork, a change project was established at the clinic, during which a leading nurse manager changed the nurse practitioners' training sessions at the hospital from being spread out across all clinics, to only one clinic (the observed clinic) in the future. In other words, the clinic would receive all the nurse practitioners from the surrounding nursing schools. The health care professionals held different opinions and interpretations of this project, some were against it and others supported it. As it turned out, the resistance or support of the change project was grounded in the values of "spending valuable time" with patients instead of "wasting time" coordinating with other health care professionals. The following presentation will therefore characterize values of spending time with patients in clinical encounters, in contrast to gathering with other health care professionals in multidisciplinary meetings, as these two everyday routines are crucial to doing and changing clinical work.

Methods: The fieldwork included observations and interviews over a six-month period. The first part included three months of observing participants' everyday lives in the ward, following day and night shifts and meetings. The strategy behind spending so much time in the ward before the interviews was to gain familiarity with the employees and their daily routines. The data concerned 20 in-depth narrative interviews with the employee groups at the ward. The narrative interviews addressed ordinary events in the everyday lives of the employees, and the employees determined all of the themes of the interviews. The opening requirement was: "Tell us about your day, from when you arrive in the morning." This interview technique served to induce storytelling (Czarniawska, 2004). Observations and daily conversations with employees were also used to help select the interview persons. The interview persons included four nurses, two social workers, an occupational therapist assigned to the ward, two patients, two ward managers, the two physiotherapists, the social counselor, a development nurse assigned to the ward, one physician, and four nurses coordinating discharge meetings with the ward on behalf of the local authorities. All of the interviews were taped and transcribed. It turned out that the narratives the health care professionals told about their patient encounters were structured narratives, with coherent, often epic plots and related to emotions and values. In contrast, the narratives told about the multidisciplinary meeting were ante-narratives, shorter and more fragmented counter-narratives, which revealed ambiguity and tensions. Thereby, an analysis of both structured and more fragmented individual narratives unfolded.[2]

Study 3: Designing Collaborative Innovation in Two Medical Wards and Collecting Policy Documents

An ethnographic study followed two local collaborative innovation projects to investigate how innovation designs were improving patient involvement in two different hospital wards. The first project was located at a breast cancer ward at a public hospital in the Capital Region of Denmark, where it was thought that the innovation project ought to improve initial medical conversations that patients have with health care professionals upon receiving a cancer diagnosis. A local health care innovation center codesigned the plans of the project processes with the ward and brought in the design elements. One design element was the introduction of patient diaries to collect patient narratives, in which patients described their experience of the initial diagnosis conversation with the staff. In workshops, the health care professions then read and discussed these diaries to gain a new sense of the patients' experiences. This project ended with the development of a novel innovation game from the innovation center to be used in all of the wards at region's hospitals to create general inspiration for innovation in the area of improving patient involvement.

The second project was located in a neurology ward at the national hospital in the capital, where the local management group hired a voluntary patient ambassador to design a new project for the ward. The aim of the project was to provide patients with feedback postcards in the waiting areas to write about their perception of their patient trajectories while being on the ward. The voluntary patient ambassador worked with a group of nurses to design, distribute, and subsequently analyze the returned postcards. Two additional external participants, a voluntary medical organization for patient safety and a large private foundation were also part of the implementation process. This collaboration resulted in the design and conceptualization of a feedback postcard, entirely funded by the foundation and the patient safety organization, for nationwide distribution for providing patient feedback.

Methods: The data in both cases in the next section derive from qualitative interviews conducted with department employees from the two wards (nurses, doctors, and clinical managers), as well as their external stakeholders. The external stakeholder interviews were conducted with the innovation consultants at the regional health innovation center and the patient ambassador. Thirty semi-structured individual interviews were conducted in total. Exclusively using a narrative interview technique (Czarniawska, 2004), informants were asked to share what they thought and felt about participating in the innovation projects. Lasting 40–80 minutes, interviews took place at the departments and in various offices. Interviews were recorded and subsequently transcribed for thematic coding and analysis. The data also included observations of meetings and innovation workshops at the hospital. At the breast cancer ward the innovation workshop was designed and facilitated by the innovation consultants. This project also included focus group interviews with patients as part of listening to them. The researcher actively participated in group work in the breast cancer workshop alongside the health care professionals. The cancer ward used the workshop to analyze the patient diaries, while the neurology ward used the meetings and a small project group to facilitate the project and analyze the findings.

The study also consisted of a historical document analysis of the public innovation policies in Denmark from 1999 to 2012. The data collection process initially began with the collection of policy documents to identify the policy narratives. First, we identified the private and public (state, regional, and local) organizations assumed to be relevant with regard to the production of policy documents involving the concept of innovation. These organizations were contacted to obtain their assistance in identifying additional policy actors and policy documents that would be particularly relevant for framing public innovation in Denmark. Using this snowball technique, data was collected until no new sources for policy documents appeared. Combined, 60 policy documents involving innovation published between 1999 and 2012 were collected. The earliest document that used the word innovation was an annual report published by the Ministry of Finance in 1999. Most of the documents collected were published from 2007 and on. A thematic analysis and NVivo software were used to analyze the data and identify the policy narratives. The policy narratives were systematically categorized based on identification of shared episodes that comprised innovation problems, solutions, and stakeholder descriptions. A policy narrative became dominant when many policy documents described the policy problem and solution in the same manner (Roe, 1997). Three dominant policy narratives emerged from the analysis.[3]

Study 4: Making Heath Care Agreements in the Regions to Coordinate Between Health Care Providers

An ethnographic study following the introduction of a national structural reform, implementing a new national regional structure replacing 13 counties with five regions by following the formation of one of the new regions and the data presented in this book are more specifically about the implementation of a health care reform (health agreements) in this region. The aim of a policy reform introducing health agreements was to coordinate patient trajectories between regions and local authorities, which are the two main public health care service sectors in Denmark, the regions being the responsible agent for hospital operations and general practice and the local authorities being the responsible agents for elderly care, social care, and rehabilitation. The health agreement was introduced in the Health Care Act and lasted two years before a new contract had to be made. The health agreements replaced health plans, which described, in detail, the region's population regarding health-related problems and challenges. The first generation of health agreements described certain areas with known coordination problems: hospital discharge processes for weak and elderly patients, including rehabilitation plans and assistive supplies, and efforts concerning mental health disorders. Each region could adjust the effort to local problems, and the health care agreements were crafted in the local health coordination committee, wherein local regional politicians, politicians from local authorities, and representatives from the union of general practitioners are members. The health care agreements had to be approved by the National Board of Health. Several ad hoc work committees were responsible for drawing up the health agreements, along with regional administrators working together with health care representatives from local authorities representing elder care, rehabilitation and social services, local GPs, and health care representatives from hospitals representing hospital wards.

Methods: The study followed the implementation of the new health care law and the introduction of health agreements through participatory observations of meeting in different committees and ad hoc committees and through qualitative interviews with politicians, administrators, and health care professionals. The interviews included both members of the National Board of Health as well as politicians and administrators at regional and municipality levels. Minutes from meetings were also collected. In total, 16 interviews were conducted with meeting participants and six meeting observations were made. The qualitative interviews were conducted using a narrative method, and exclusively using a narrative interview technique (Czarniawska, 2004); informants were asked to share what they thought and felt about participating in the meetings. Most of the interviews and meeting observations were conducted in the early days of the implementation and at the beginning of the process of making the agreements after the new law was in effect. Lasting 60–70 minutes, interviews took place at regional town halls, where most of the meetings were held. Interviews were recorded and subsequently transcribed for thematic coding and analysis. As this analysis was part of a larger project about the formation of a new region, the data was supplemented by general qualitative interviews of all regional politicians and top executives, conducted by other researchers in the project.[4]

The data in these projects was collected without any kind of requirements or restrictions attached from the funders' side. They all involved following the everyday life of the people working in the organizations, and they represent a collection of field studies illustrating organizational change processes during everyday organizing.

The Order of Chapters

After the introduction, the second chapter presents the theoretical background: the narrative framework of the book, while the last chapter discusses the findings from the intervening chapters and answers the research questions asked in this introduction. The analytical chapters in this volume (3–7) refer to the four organizational ethnographic studies just presented. The first part of each chapter provides a theoretical presentation of the organizational phenomena the chapter is about, while the second part presents the empirical findings to not only support the theoretical section but also to expand it.

Chapter 2. A Theoretical Narrative Approach to Organizational Change Studies

In this chapter a narrative approach will be presented combining narratives, arguing that both structured and more provisory narratives are useful in studies of change and innovation processes because they both have the capacity to direct new sense and make sense of everyday organizing. The fragmented, or ante- (pre-), narratives are often told as contradictory narratives with tensions, ambiguity, and discontinuity as sensemaking processes (Boje, 2001; Cunliffe, Luhman, & Boje, 2004; Vaara et al., 2016). The structured narratives are defined by a chain of events directed by a plot or causal relationships between the events and are often told to persuade others to follow an idea and to create shared sensemaking processes (Gabriel, 2000; Pedersen & Johansen, 2012).

Chapter 3. Making Sense of Everyday Innovation at a Clinical Ward Through Narratives of Visitation Routines

The purpose of this chapter is to demonstrate the sensemaking condition of a local organizational change processes in a hospital ward. The field study is about the introduction of a new visitation triage model at an emergency ward. The theoretical section presents theories on organizational change and everyday innovation. Organizational change is a classical theme in organizational studies. As Chapter 2 states, a narrative approach to organizational change consists of the change participants' various perceptions of change and views change processes as sensemaking processes, which never cease, as change in organizations is continuous (Weick & Quinn, 1999).

The second part of the chapter presents findings from the study of an emergency ward. A clinical manager came up with the idea of introducing a new triage visitation model to prioritize patients in a more standardized way. The clinical manager's strategic spokesperson narrative of the change idea is presented first, followed by a presentation of the ante-narratives of health care professionals as they talked about how they understood working with the new visitation routine. Last, a patient's illness narrative is presented. Shared while she was waiting on the ward, it describes her understanding of the visitation routine. Together these narratives provide a picture of the polyphonic conditions of organizational change processes in health care organizations. Change and organizing do not always happen based on shared or collective understandings, hence, new routines in everyday life are understood based on diverse voices, deriving from both the structured and fragmented individual narratives of clinical managers, health care professionals, and patients.

Chapter 4. A Resistance and Everyday View on Health Care Professionals

The purpose of this chapter is to understand the values of health care professionals and their potential resistance toward change processes in a rehabilitation ward. The first section describes concepts from a theory of professions. Evetts (2003) wrote that most analyses of professionalism, as a normative value system, have been at macro- and meso-levels of analysis (p. 399). In contrast to this, the focus on everyday organizing in hospital wards is, per se, a micro-level focus on health care professionals, including different groups of health care professionals, e.g., nurses, physicians, therapists, medical assistants, and midwives.

In the second part of the chapter two types of narratives by the health care professionals are presented, reflecting everyday routines of health care professionals and patients. The first type of narrative concerns the clinical encounter, where the reflections of the professionals revolve around their relationships to patients and how these relationships help form their professional values. The second part of the analysis presents narratives from multidisciplinary meetings, demonstrating how professionals collaborate with each other based on mutual understanding that is formed in professional groups. The narrative analyses examined both structured narratives and more fragmented narratives, making it possible to understand both the strong values of health care professionals formulated in more structured narratives, where they talk about their values regarding patient interactions, and the struggle and tensions between their duty to professional groups, told more as counter-narratives and ante-narratives. This analysis contributes by describing which local values influence the health care professionals' interpretations and narratives.

Chapter 5. Designing and Driving Collaborative, Everyday Innovation Using Narratives

The purpose of this chapter is to examine how innovative design thinking from the innovation literature mobilized participants in two local collaborative innovation projects. The first part of the chapter describes core concepts from the collaborative innovation literature, including external stakeholder participation that can solve complex problems. The underlining innovation assumption is that a disruption of everyday routines brought about by the introduction of new external voices, for example patient voices, is a design method that would be useful to innovate.

The second part presents narratives from the two collaborative innovation projects, beginning with the shared narratives of the health care professionals and clinical managers that support shared local values and mobilization of participants in the projects. Next, individual ante-narratives by patients and participants are presented to illustrate how new sensemaking is emerging about patient values. The contribution of this chapter is to illustrate how two shared narratives can redirect the sensemaking of heath care professions and other external participants concerning everyday routines involving waiting time and medical consultations. The analysis also shows how individual ante-narratives both can be positive or critical towards innovative design thinking.

Chapter 6. Organizational Change Through Narratives of Administrative Coordination

The purpose of this chapter is to demonstrate the sensemaking conditions of coordination efforts in health agreements between regions and local authorities, where coordination is seen as an administrative, top-down condition for organizational change. The need for coordination is an example of an administrative change condition leading to new ways of coordinating. The first, theoretical, part of the chapter describes traditional strands of organizational theories of coordination, which are based on the assumption that coordination is the outcome of processes within coherent, institutionally, or functionally demarcated units that follow a specific, pre-given, rational logic of consequentiality. In recent years a unitary understanding of coordination has been challenged by a more pluricentric understanding.

The second part of the chapter presents three shared narratives by politicians and administrators in their efforts to draw up new health care agreements on coordination. The first one deals with secure operations, the second involves equal partnerships, and the third narrative is about control. The contribution of this chapter is that it demonstrates how sensemaking becomes a central condition of coordination between regions and the local authorities because the three shared narratives create new, legitimate, and illegitimate ways of coordinating.

Chapter 7. Policy Narratives of Innovation Expectations

The purpose of this chapter is to illuminate how public policy ideas on change and innovation translate into policy narratives and describe policy expectations concerning how to organize innovative health care organizations. Policy narratives are examples of political change conditions, revealing examples of legitimate ways of becoming innovative. The first part of the chapter describes three dominant public management perspectives of the last 20 years: traditional public administration, new public management, and network governance.

The second part of this chapter describes three policy narratives, identified based on an analysis of policy documents on public innovation. The narratives describe how innovation should be obtained in a new partnerships model through public research infrastructure that supports private innovation and also by innovative welfare employees. This chapter adds to our understanding of organizational narratives by illustrating how they relate to other types of narratives, in this case, policy narratives. The everyday organizing context also relates to a dynamic policy context, as policy narratives about innovation are inspired by different public management ideas. In some ways, they affect the societal expectations of becoming an innovative health care organization.

The overall conclusion from the analytical chapters, moving from an individual, to an organizational to a policy view of change processes, is to demonstrate how organizational everyday ethnographies can occur by bridging theoretical discussions of organizational change concepts: routines, resistance, innovation, coordination, and public management, with empirical findings and narratives from situated change processes. Thus presenting a picture of the central role of frontline workers, their work, their narratives, and their sensemaking in situated change processes, where every day organizing and its relation to other types of organizing becomes part of organizational change processes.

Notes

1. This study was partly funded by a local hospital and a research assistant was part of the project. The research assistant, Mette Brehm Johansen, conducted the field studies. Some of the findings presented in Chapter 3 are also published in: Johansen, M. B. (2010). Innovation og triagearbejde-en kvalitativ undersøgelse af triage på Akutafdelingen, Hillerød Hospital. *Center for Health Management, Copenhagen Business school, Copenhagen*, 1–66; Pedersen, A. R., & Johansen, M. B. (2012). Strategic and everyday innovative narratives: Translating ideas into everyday life in organizations. *The Innovation Journal*, 17(1), 2. I thank Mette Brehm Johansen for an always inspiring collaboration.
2. This project was funded by the university and involved hiring a research assistant. The researcher, together with the research assistant, conducted the data collection. Some of the findings presented in Chapter 4 are also published in Pedersen, A. R. (2008). Narrative identity work in a medical ward: A study of diversity in health care identities. *Tamara: Journal for Critical Organization Inquiry*, 7(1).
3. This project was funded by the strategic research council and was part of a larger research project on collaborative innovation in public organizations. A student assistant performed part of the document analysis. Parts of the findings are published in Pedersen, A. R. (2016). The role of patient narratives in health care innovation: Supporting translation and meaning making. *Journal of Health Organization and Management*, 30(2), 244–257; Pedersen, A. R. (2013). Collaborative narrative innovation: A case of public innovation in Denmark. In A. Andreas Müller & L. Lutz Becker (Eds.), *Narrative and innovation: New ideas for business administration, strategic management and entrepreneurship* (pp. 57–65). Wiesbaden: Springer VS; Pedersen, A. R. (2015). Organizational healthcare innovation performed by contextual sense making. In E. Ferlie, S. Boch Waldorff, A. Reff Pedersen, L. Fitzgerald, & P. G. Lewis (Eds.), *Managing change: From health policy to practice* (pp. 238–253). London: Palgrave Macmillan. Susanne Boch Waldorff was an inspiring research colleague to work with, thanks.
4. This project was part of a larger research project about the formation of a new region funded by the public taxation foundation. Several researchers were part of interviewing the administrators and politicians in the region. Some of the findings in Chapter 6 are also published in Pedersen, A. R., Sehested, K., & Sørensen, E. (2011). Emerging theoretical understanding of pluricentric coordination in public governance. *The American Review of Public Administration*, 41(4), 375–394. I would like to thank Eva Sørensen and Karina Sehested for our inspiring, ongoing discussions.

References

Akrich, M., Callon, M., Latour, B., & Monaghan, A. (2002). The key to success in innovation part I: The art of interessement. *International Journal of Innovation Management*, 6(02), 187–206.

Allen, D. (2002). *The changing shape of nursing practice: The role of nurses in the hospital division of labour*. New York and London: Routledge.

Bartel, C. A., & Garud, R. (2009). The role of narratives in sustaining organizational innovation. *Organization Science, 20*(1), 107–117.

Boje, D. M. (2001). *Narrative methods for organizational & communication research*. Thousand Oaks, CA: Sage.

Borum, F. (1995). The unprepared journey into the hospital world. In I. Andersen, F. Brum, P. Kristensen, & P. Karnøe (Eds.), *On the art of doing field studies* (pp. 61–85). Frederiksberg: Handelshøjskolens Forlag.

Bruner, J. (1991). The narrative construction of reality. *Critical Inquiry, 18*(1), 1–21.

Cunliffe, A. L., Luhman, J. T., & Boje, D. M. (2004). Narrative temporality: Implications for organizational research. *Organization Studies, 25*(2), 261–286.

Czarniawska, B. (1997). *Narrating the organization: Dramas of institutional identity*. Chicago, IL: University of Chicago Press.

Czarniawska, B. (2004). *Narratives in social science research*. London: Sage.

Czarniawska-Joerges, B. (2007). *Shadowing and other techniques for doing fieldwork in modern societies*. Copenhagen, Denmark: Copenhagen Business School Press.

Evetts, J. (2003). The sociological analysis of professionalism: Occupational change in the modern world. *International Sociology, 18*(2), 395–415.

Ferlie, E. (2016). *Analysing health care organizations*. London: Routledge.

Ferlie, E., Fitzgerald, L., Wood, M., & Hawkins, C. (2005). The nonspread of innovations: The mediating role of professionals. *Academy of Management Journal, 48*(1), 117–134.

Ferlie, E., Montgomery, K., & Pedersen, A. R. (Eds.). (2016). *The Oxford handbook of health care management*. London: Oxford University Press.

Foucault, M. (1973a). *The birth of the clinic*. London: Tavistock.

Foucault, M. (1973b). *The birth of the clinic: An archaeology of medical perception* (A. M. Sheridan Smith, Trans.). New York, NY: Pantheon.

Gabriel, Y. (2000). *Storytelling in organizations: Facts, fictions, and fantasies*. London: Oxford University Press.

Goffman, E. (1968). *Asylums: Essays on the social situation of mental patients and other inmates*. Piscataway, NJ: Aldine Transaction.

Hammersley, M., & Atkinson, P. (2007). *Ethnography: Principles in practice*. London: Routledge.

Hernes, T. (2014). *A process theory of organization*. London: Oxford University Press.

Johansen, M. B. (2010). Innovation og triagearbejde-en kvalitativ undersøgelse af triage på Akutafdelingen, Hillerød Hospital. Center for Health Management, Copenhagen Business School, Copenhagen, 1–66

McDermott, A. M., & Pedersen, A. R. (2016). Conceptions of patients and their roles in healthcare: Insights from everyday practice and service improvement. *Journal of Health Organization and Management, 30*(2), 194–206.

Mol, A. (2002). *The body multiple: Ontology in medical practice*. Durham, NC; and London: Duke University Press.

Nickelsen, N. C. M. (2019). The infrastructure of telecare: Implications for nursing tasks and the nurse-doctor relationship. *Sociology of Health & Illness, 41*(1), 67–80.

Neyland, D. (2007). *Organizational ethnography*. London: Sage.

Pedersen, A. R. (2008). Narrative identity work in a medical ward: A study of diversity in health care identities. *Tamara: Journal for Critical Organization Inquiry, 7*(1).

Pedersen, A. R. (2009). Moving away from chronological time: Introducing the shadows of time and chronotopes as new understandings of narrative time. *Organization, 16*(3), 389–406.

Pedersen, A. R., & Johansen, M. B. (2012). Strategic and everyday innovative narratives: Translating ideas into everyday life in organizations. *The Innovation Journal, 17*(1), 2.

Pedersen, A. R., Sehested, K., & Sørensen, E. (2011). Emerging theoretical understanding of pluricentric coordination in public governance. *The American Review of Public Administration, 41*(4), 375–394.

Pedersen, A. R., & Humle, D. M. (Eds.). (2016). *Doing organizational ethnography: A focus on polyphonic ways of organizing*. London: Routledge.

Pope, C. (2005). Conducting ethnography in medical settings. *Medical Education, 39*(12), 1180–1187.

Reay, T., & Hinings, C. R. (2009). Managing the rivalry of competing institutional logics. *Organization Studies, 30*(6), 629–652.

Scott, W. R., Ruef, M., Mendel, P. J., & Caronna, C. A. (2000). *Institutional change and healthcare organizations: From professional dominance to managed care*. Chicago, IL: University of Chicago Press.

Turner, B. S. (1983). *Medical power and social knowledge*. London: Sage.

Vaara, E., Sonenshein, S., & Boje, D. (2016). Narratives as sources of stability and change in organizations: Approaches and directions for future research. *Academy of Management Annals, 10*(1), 495–560.

Weick, K. E., & Quinn, R. E. (1999). Organizational change and development. *Annual Review of Psychology, 50*(1), 361–386.

Ybema, S., Yanow, D., Wels, H., & Kamsteeg, F. H. (Eds.). (2009). *Organizational ethnography: Studying the complexity of everyday life*. London: Sage.

2 A Theoretical Narrative Approach to Organizational Change Studies

Why is the study of narratives important in organizational change studies? Should narratives be reserved for folkloric bedtime storytelling for children? No narratives are a single kind of conversation that happens in organizations every day. People in organizations talk—they make sense of their talks and they reject ideas that make no sense to them. Organizational change processes are conditioned in the sense they create for the participants involved, and one way to understand the possibilities of change is to investigate how change processes affect our understanding of change and organizing. The main assumption about organizational change using a narrative approach is that, if people do not understand the need for change, they will have a tendency to reject it. They need to understand the meaning of change to make it happen. Thereby, organizational change is intertwined with the sensemaking of the participants involved regarding the intentions and events of the change.

The purpose of this chapter is to unfold a framework of multiple narrative theories and present the possibilities of working with narratives in studies of organizational change and innovation. Common to all the narrative theories presented in this chapter is that they represent an interpretative narrative approach dealing with narrative constructions as the object of study. Both individual narratives and shared narratives will be presented, demonstrating how change processes are both effects of sensemaking by *individual narratives* and capture the collective sensemaking of a group of people in *shared narratives*. Thereby, organizational narratives can include both individual or personal narratives, helping individuals to make sense, and shared or composite narratives representing collective meanings.

The first part of this chapter presents narratives as sensemaking conditions in organizational change processes. The second part presents the threefold narrative framework and discusses the possibilities of using this framework in everyday ethnographic studies of organizational change.

Narratives as Sensemaking Conditions in Organizational Change Processes

This section presents how narratives are linked to sensemaking processes in organizational change processes and how this book defines narratives.

Barbara Czarniawska, Yiannis Gabriel, and David Boje are three of the early scholars of narrative studies in organizations. Czarniawska (2004) points out that organizing is intertwined with narratives, as people in organizations make interpretations of what is going on through narratives. They represent different narrative approaches, as they are inspired by a blend of narrative sources in human and social sciences. They are, for example, a philosophical and literature approach (Bakhtin, 1981; Brooks, 1992; MacIntyre, 1988; Polkinghorne, 1988); a folkloristic, psychological, or sociological approach (Bruner, 1990; Frye, 1957; Gubrium & Holstein, 1998; Mishler, 2004); and an organizational approach (Brown, Gabriel, & Gherardi, 2009; Garud, Dunbar, & Bartel, 2011; Georges, 1980; Martin, 1983; Tsoukas, 2005; Van Maanen, 1988). As the early scholars are inspired by a blend of these narrative strands and resources, the theoretical approaches in this book also draw inspiration from these directions, combining philosophical, psychological, and organizational narrative theories.

The word sensemaking used in this book does not address sensemaking processes from a Weick (1995) perspective or from the organizational literature on sensemaking (Balogun, Bartunek, & Do, 2015; Lockett, Currie, Finn, Martin, & Waring, 2014; Maitlis & Christianson, 2014; Sonenshein, 2010), asserting that sensemaking occurs in relation to particular cognitive frames or enactments. Instead, sensemaking is a social and relational process and a narrative approach does not argue that specific organizing actions or contexts lead to collective or individual sensemaking. This narrative approach follows the simple arguments of Bruner (1990), that people tell stories to make sense. Consequently, sensemaking becomes a relational, performative phenomena, whereas telling is as important as the final narrative. People do not tell stories out of the blue; they relate to culturally accepted ways of telling, which means that Western narratives are different from other cultural traditions and values, as narratives reflect our cultural values and already culturally accepted forms of narratives (Bruner, 1990).

Narratives are told for a reason; they are told to make sense. Bruner (1990) interpreted the function of narrating in a dramaturgical sense, stating, "when we enter human life it is as if we walk on stage into a play whose enactment is already in progress . . . a play whose somewhat open plot determines what parts we may play and toward what denouements we may be heading" (p. 33). Hence, narratives direct our interpretations. Bruner also had an explanation of the functions of a story, which is to find an intentional state that migrates, or at least makes comprehensive, a deviation from a canonical cultural pattern (p. 49). In that way we use narratives to understand what is going on in our lives, and to understand what is perceived as normal or deviant behavior.

In the past 30 years, narratives have been a widely used theoretical lens and method for studying organizational change in organizations (Cunliffe & Coupland, 2012; Currie & Brown, 2003; Dailey & Browning, 2014; Downing, 1997; Feldman, Sköldberg, Brown, & Horner, 2004; Gabriel, 1995; Pedersen, 2009; Rhodes & Brown, 2005; Sonenshein, 2010; Vaara, 2002). Vaara, Sonenshein, and Boje (2016) argued that the continued use of narrative in organizational and management studies reflects their utility and versatility. In a study of managers and their sensemaking of success and failure in a post-merger organizational change process, Vaara (2002) identified four types of narrative discourses that attributed either blame or responsibility of the change processes: rationalistic, cultural, role-bound, and individualistic. Sonenshein (2010) studied how people responded and made interpretations of strategic change through three types of narratives—progressive, stability, or regressive narratives—while Reissner (2011) found that individual narratives of organizational change were told in three different ways to understand the change events: as the good old days, as deception, taboo, and silence, or as influence. Last, Rhodes, Pullen, and Clegg (2010) described a narrative of organizational change in a technological company as the inevitable, fall-from-grace narration, portraying a narrative of an organization whose destiny is to decline. These recent narrative organizational change studies point to three different narrative conditions of organizational change: the relations between the narratives themselves and organizational sensemaking, the polyphonic sensemaking condition (including alternative meanings/counter-narratives), and the relation between interpretations of change and interpretations of cultural values and representation of ethics.

Defining Organizational Narratives

In this book, the word "narratives" means the final narrative product, and storytelling refers to processes of telling narratives. In some studies, stories and narratives are used interchangeably, but in this book, "narratives" is used to avoid unnecessary complexity.

The word "narratives," which is an important concept in narrative approaches in organizational studies and in the various types of narrative studies, is represented by many definitions of narratives or storytelling, but common to all studies is the premise that narratives are part of making sense of our lives, as they are a part of making sense of our everyday work and life in organizations.

Vaara et al. (2016) defined narratives broadly as temporal, discursive constructions that provide a means for individual, social, and organizational sensemaking and sense giving (p. 3). This means that their constructions can vary, and they can be analyzed on multiple analytical levels, from micro- to macro-levels. This definition stresses the role of temporal, discursive, sensemaking, and sense giving processes in organizations. They further underlined how organizational narratives can provide an essential means for maintaining or reproducing stability and/or promoting resistance to change in and around organizations (p. 4).

Vaara et al. (2016) further described how organizational narrative studies take three approaches to organizational change: a realist approach, where narrative represents data; an interpretative approach, where narratives are conceptualized as the individual's constructions of organizational phenomena; and last, a poststructuralist approach, where narrative deconstruction demonstrates how dominant narratives often are problematized (p. 15). The narrative approach that is used in the following chapters in this book is an interpretative one, wherein the focus is on the description and elaboration of narratives that play a central role in the social construction of organizational reality. Some of the subsequent chapters present individual narratives addressing the polyphonic sensemaking conditions of narratives and storytelling in change processes, while others present shared or composite narratives, which capture collective meanings of groups of participants. Both types of interpretative narratives provide an important window into the multiple meanings of stability and change, as Vaara et al. (2016) noted that organizational narratives have the capacity to reveal alternative meanings that impact change that may otherwise go unnoticed (p. 21).

In this book, narratives are explained via a threefold narrative framework as: structured narratives, fragmented ante-narratives, or combined structured and fragmented narratives. Structured narratives represent a classical way of understanding narratives through the coherent relations between characters, events, and plots (Gabriel, 2000), and ante-narratives represent a more critical tradition, wherein narratives can create sensemaking without a causality of events (Boje, 2008). The basis for using a combined model is that both structured and fragmented narratives *should* be included in narrative analysis (Bartel & Garud, 2009). By including these three definitions of narratives, this book builds on a pragmatic narrative tradition, with inspiration from Bartel and Garud (2009), arguing for including both structured and provisory narratives in our understanding of organizational narratives

In relation to the presented definition of Vaara et al.'s (2016) narratives, which related narratives to discourse, temporal constructions, and sensemaking and sense giving, this book defines organizational narratives as: *structured and fragmented interpretative social constructions that provide means for both individual and collective sensemaking.* This definition includes narratives as phenomena related to storytellers or authors and both a temporal/time narrative perspective (Vaara & Pedersen, 2013; Pedersen, 2009). A more Weick (1995) sensemaking/sense giving perspective (Sonenshein, 2010) is not included in this definition, although these narrative traditions are also interesting and relevant to investigate further in future research on organizational change. Instead, the focus is on the assorted types of organizational narratives that create sense of organizational change processes.

Partial Discussion and Conclusion

A common feature of the ethnography studies presented in the next chapters is that they show how organizational change relate to the narratives of the participants in change processes, e.g., patients, health care professionals, clinical managers, and external collaborators, not because they are the only important people in organizational change processes. Instead of analyzing general sensemaking processes, the pragmatic narrative framework has the ability to explain which participants become involved in creating locally situated sensemaking of change processes.

Furthermore, the narrative framework also has the ability to illustrate the specific change intentions and change events that evolve sensemaking in an everyday, situated context. As the next chapter will present, organizational change processes are often driven from local units, i.e., from clinical wards, where patients, health care professionals, and clinical managers make sense of and participate in various local change projects.

A Combined Narrative Framework

The individual and shared narratives presented in the next part of the chapter are defined in three different ways, as they can present as *structured narratives, fragmented narratives*, or as *combined fragmented and structured narratives*. A coherent plot of events defines structured narratives, and the lack of a coherent plot of events defines fragmented narratives. Both individual and shared/composite narratives can be expressed by structured and fragmented narratives. Currie and Brown (2003) conducted a study of a hospital and created a narrative not articulated by one individual but by many, formed as fragments. This threefold narrative framework represents a pragmatic narrative view by including coexisting narrative definitions. The argument of choosing this narrative framework is that when doing an everyday ethnography the ethnographer meets many different narratives in and around organizations, some told in a more intentional, structured manner, and others told in a more fragmented, critical manner as counternarratives. The sum of these different individual and shared narratives, together or separately, provides a polyphonic picture of sensemaking and change processes.

A Structural Narrative Approach

The structural narrative approaches presented here were inspired by the narrative studies of Gabriel (2000) that explored the idea of narratives and how they may be used as an interpretive device in trying to understand the interaction between managers and employees, and how they make sense of everyday organizational life. Gabriel (2000) defined organizational stories as types of sensemaking devices that focus on storytelling in a narrow sense, with simple but resonant plots and characters that involve narrative skills, poetic tropes, and taking risks, all of which are combined to entertain, persuade, and win over (p. 22). According to Gabriel, narratives are poetic modes of storytelling. Inspired by Canadian literary critic and theorist, Northrup Frye's (1957) work with myths and archetypes, Gabriel defined four narrative genres (p. 84), which are listed in Table 2.1

Table 2.1 defines how an epic or heroic story focuses on the valiant character and agency and brave achievements in particular, such as missions or crisis resolution (Gabriel, 2000, p. 74). The predominant emotions are pride and admiration. In contrast to the epic story, the tragic story casts the protagonist as the victim and makes feelings such as grief, pain, fear, anger, and shame central. The victims bring about their own downfall through their own actions and destiny, and the key poetic trope is the attribution of blame to a supernatural principle, such as fate or a malevolent agent (Gabriel, 2000, p. 70). The plots of romantic stories, the third narrative genre, revolve around romantic love and tokens of love, gratitude, and appreciation. Gabriel (2000) found many romantic stories at hospitals, wherein staff talked about grateful patients who bring them chocolates or cards. The stories showed compassion for patients and colleagues (p. 80). The last genre, comic stories, occurs when the protagonist

Table 2.1 Four Narrative Genres

	Epic	Tragic	Romantic	Comic
PROTAGONIST CHARACTERS	Hero, Villain, Rescue object	Victim, Helper, Villain	Love object Gift giver, Lover	Fool Trickster
PLOT FOCUS AND POETIC TROPES	Achievement, noble victory, contest, agency	Undeserved misfortune, loss, crime, malevolent fate	Love triumphant, recognition, emotions	Misfortune as deserved, mistake, providential significance
EMOTIONS	Pride, nostalgia, admiration	Sorrow, pity, fear	Love, care	Hate, scorn

Source of inspiration: Gabriel (2000)

is a survivor, a humorist, or an ironist. The teller of these stories rejects self-pity but refuses to capitulate while stopping short of rebellion or confrontation (Gabriel, 2000, p. 65). Gabriel points out that many hybrid stories are made up of these combinations of stories: romantic/comic, tragic/comic, and epic/romantic. Gabriel related the narrative genres to the storytelling he collected in organizational fields. His aim was to collect many types of stories and to demonstrate the variety and the connection between storytelling, emotions, trust, and poetic modes.

Sköldberg (1994) and Downing (1997) provided two examples of the analysis of organizational change using a structural narrative approach. Sköldberg analyzed organizational change in a Swedish local government organization and focused on how people experienced change as expressed in their narrative accounts. He identified four narrative genres: tragedy, romantic, comedy, and satire. He concluded that the narrative condition formed the meaning of the changes for the people involved. Downing's (1997) study addressed how organizational change evoked a period of emotional and interpretative conflicts that shareholders resolved by sharing stories about unfolding events and by identifying the plots of change. He identified four plots of organizational change: the quest, a progressive hero adventure; the downfall, a hero is pitched from success to danger and humiliation; the contest, a polarized struggle between two heroes; and, last, the scam, wherein the hero is exposed as incompetent, corrupt, or a fool (Downing, 1997, p. 37). Downing ended by arguing that leaders in organizations attempt to frame organizational change as a romantic quest, which approximates the literary form of fulfilling a dream (Frye, 1957, p. 186 in Downing, 1997, p. 40) and expressing feelings of satisfaction. Downing's study also demonstrated how feelings such as sadness, anger, or fear also can be enacted to make sense of organizational dramas in change processes. The structural approach thus invites us to relate organizational change processes not only to individual feelings and emotions but also to the shared structured narratives that can be found in organizational change processes that direct collective sensemaking processes (see Chapters 5 and 6).

A Fragmented, Ante-Narrative Approach

Recent studies of organizational narratives suggest that narratives are not to be conceived as stable structures; stories are not isolated elements. In this approach, the concepts of stories and story work are used, pointing to the fragmented nature of narratives and enhancing a processual and performative view on narratives.

Boje's (1991, 1995, 2008) narrative research has been at the forefront of the fragmented narrative view in organizational and management studies. Boje's main point is that organizational stories are not isolated phenomena; they become part of other stories, integrating and mingling with them. He (1991) has focused on how individual stories become a part of the collective mental landscape of the organization through ongoing interactive processes within the organization. In these interactive processes, stories meet and change in the permanent act of storytelling through power games between competing stories. He further investigated this theme through the definition of ante-narratives as fragmented stories without a plot, pointing out how stories reflect the organizations in which they exist. Emerging and dynamic organizational forms, for instance, create incomplete stories because "people are only tracing story fragments, inventing bits and pieces to glue it all together, but never able to visit all the stages and see the whole" (Boje, 2001, p. 5). Organizational ante-narratives often differ from structured narratives, as they are often oral and highly colored by the organizational context in which they are told.

Fragmented narrative studies frequently direct attention to the storyteller and the narrative practice with which the narratives are made. In a study of a company supply office, Boje (1991) described five storytelling features related to the narrator. First, attempts are made to negotiate different interpretations into a story with one plot. Second, the details of a story depend on whether or not the audience already knows the story. Third, storytelling rights will vary, i.e., some storytellers will have certain rights depending on experience, persuasive abilities, and status. Fourth, there are also storytellers with a varying capacity to tell stories. Some are good at performing a story with passion and affection, while others are less competent. Finally, some stories can seem legitimate to tell if they are related to already accepted discourses, e.g., how new public management affects hospitals. In sum, Boje points out how the narrators, beyond the narrative itself, are an important part of performing a story as story work.

Gubrium and Holstein (1998) also put emphasis on this focus on storytelling processes as narrative practice. They defined stories as narrative practice, which means that stories are told in the context of certain institutionalized cultural settings. Personal accounts reflect experience and, therefore, personal storytelling is defined as the interplay of discursive actions and the circumstances of storytelling (p. 164). In this way, storytellers are not merely communicative puppets of their circumstances but provide personal accounts created based on their experience and preferred vocabularies. A main condition of fragmented narratives is the lack of coherence. In support of Mishler's (2004) critique of the search for coherence in stories, the partial presence and absence of coherence in stories must be identified, a process that can arguably be unfolded by focusing on different forms of fragmentation in narratives (Humle & Pedersen, 2014).

One type of fragmentation is discontinuities, which Mishler (2004) defined as unresolved identity dilemmas, pointing out how stories are often improvised and how the creative potential of interrupted and conflicted lives can be explored by studying diversity and ambiguity (p. 14). In contrast to continuity, discontinuity means that stories are not told in a logical sequence of events (e.g., she gets a degree and then a job); instead, stories are told with a lack of coherence and describe numerous events in a variety of tenses. Another type of fragmentation is created by tensions (Mishler, 2004), which are not dichotomous but the result of multiple perspectives, wherein several stories are told at once and the storytelling contains ambiguity and uncertainty. Consequently, tensions become a natural part of storytelling in the search for coherence and are thus co-constructed processes that illustrate multiple perspectives. Narrative editing, the last example of fragmentation, is a concept that highlights the reflexive agency of the storyteller. The storyteller needs to share their story from a perspective and is constantly involved in monitoring, managing, modifying, and revising the story work (Gubrium & Holstein, 1998, p. 170). As a result, the role of editing is to create a specific perception of the storyteller by placing the story in a time and space and by selecting perspective and relationships involved in the events described. Two types of editing are narrative linkage and slippages. They negotiate the ways in which stories are linked together through editing and how stories are connected, assembled, rearranged, and revised in relation to coping with discontinuities (p. 167). Elasticity is created in stories through gaps and links between different cultural categories in which cultural resources provide material for the narrator to construct their own story. Table 2.2 shows the three types of narrative fragmentation.

In a narrative fragmentation approach, storytelling and story work is an ongoing process. The previously mentioned studies share an understanding of how sensemaking is not bound to a rationality or causality and coherence of events but also happens during the fragmented storytelling process. The studies demonstrate how the practice of storytelling functions by editing, assembling, negotiating, and controlling stories to cope with the tensions and discontinuities of telling narratives.

Table 2.2 Types of Narrative Fragmentation

	Narrative practice	*Sensemaking in story work*
DISCONTINUITY	Ambiguity and complexity	Blurred stories and ambiguity
TENSIONS	Multiple and diverse perspectives	Different layers of stories and sensemaking
EDITING	Linkages, gaps, slippages	Self-editing as a processes of making sense

Source of inspiration: Humle & Pedersen, 2014

Recent studies describe fragmented narratives of tensions as counter-narratives, which are "stories which people tell and live which offer resistance, either implicitly or explicitly, to dominant cultural narratives" (Frandsen, Kuhn, & Lundholt, 2016, p. 2). This means that they are always related to other, more established narratives. Consequently, counter-narratives are communicated in less structured and more incomplete terms than structured narratives, without a plot, events, and characters, but rather as ante-narratives.

Recent studies of organizational change from a fragmented narrative approach often illustrate the alternative voices, the silent voice, or the counter-narratives in organizational change processes. In their study of change processes in a public sector collaboration, Fronda and Moriceau (2008) found how resistance to change can be a safeguard toward an over-optimistic view of change. They also demonstrated the confrontation between grand narratives and ante-narratives. In another study of ante-narratives of organizational change, Boje, Harley, and Saylors (2016) studied an international burger restaurant, its strategizing, and how ante-narratives highlighted emergent conflicts and their resolution for sensemaking, which included diverse organizational stakeholders and influenced organizational effectiveness. Together, these studies demonstrate how the struggle over meanings occurs in change processes and how stabilizing narratives are challenged by ante-narratives and counter-narratives, resulting in a limitation of the value of strategic narratives of change.

A Combined Narrative Approach

The last approach combines both structured and fragmented narratives. A narrative and organizational study by Bartel and Garud (2009) demonstrated how innovation narratives are both structured and provisionary and that both traits aid coordination in processes of innovation. They defined two kinds of innovation narratives: structured narratives, which have plots and coherence, and provisory narratives, which have a fragmented structure and show that aspects are an important part of innovation processes. Both types of narrative stress the relationships and knowledge in organizations. In the health care innovation literature, Pedersen and Johansen (2012) investigated the need to include both strategically structured spokesperson narratives and more fragmented inter-professional ante-narratives. Innovation ideas are implemented to allow health care professionals to be skeptical and to express positive and negative feelings toward the innovative practices. As such, narratives can express and create strategic goals and future directions, as well as oppose, counter, and resist them by expressing different meanings on a shared issue.

The combining narrative approach represents a pragmatically applied narrative understanding, taking its departure from the point of view wherein both structured and fragmented narratives can be found in and around organizations. This is not arguing for one way of defining narratives but allowing for a more inclusive approach, which allows multiple organizationally situated local contexts to define the empirical found narratives. Thereby this approach fits well with the use of organizational ethnography, wherein field studies and the inclusion of different qualitative methods interact with the theoretical approach, without deductive definitions of narratives beforehand.

Conclusion and Discussion

This chapter presented a narrative approach to organizational change. By introducing three different ways of using a narrative analysis (structured, fragmented, and combined) to understand the various conditions involved in organizational change processes, we acknowledge the history and development of narrative contributions.

Table 2.3 summarizes the narrative approaches that will be used in the following chapters.

These narrative approaches each contribute differently to the sensemaking of change. Combined, the narrative framework's various approaches stress how organizational change processes are conditioned by culturally accepted ways of telling stories of change but also demonstrate how ongoing negotiations of storytelling are part of change processes and how dominant, more fragmented narratives are part of the understandings of change. Finally, the narrative framework also identifies the work change participants undertake when telling narratives or doing story work, a

Table 2.3 Three Different Approaches to Narrative Analysis

	Structured narratives	Fragmented narratives	Combined approaches
CORE CONCEPTS	Characters, plot focus, and emotions	Discontinuities, tensions, editing	Structured and provisory narratives
ANALYTICAL CONCEPTS	Epic, tragic romantic, and comic narratives	Ambiguity, multiple layers, linkages, gaps, and slippages	Spokespersons' narratives and counter-narratives
SENSEMAKING	Dominant narratives of events and plots	Fragmentation in negotiations of story work	Relations between different kinds of narratives

condition researchers often leave out, imagining narratives as final products. In this framework, organizational narratives are social constructions, negotiating values of right and wrong, often illustrating the unseen consequences of organizational change processes.

To conclude, a narrative approach to organizational change contributes with knowledge of how people tell narratives in their work life in organizations. They tell stories to make sense of change ideas, strategies, or events in relation to their everyday contexts and in relation to their values. Their narratives reflect normal ways of sharing narratives in their local contexts. Organizational change happens by redirecting sensemaking, but a great deal of effort is involved in changing sensemaking. This approach is only relevant in organizational change processes in which change events evoke sensemaking. The narrative analysis can demonstrate how resistance, engagement, participation, and coordination are all sensemaking-related activities and valuable narratives for generating change ideas, strategies, and events.

References

Bakhtin, M. M. (1981). *The dialogic imagination: Four essays by M. M. Bakhtin.* Austin, TX: University of Texas Press.

Balogun, J., Bartunek, J. M., & Do, B. (2015). Senior managers' sensemaking and responses to strategic change. *Organization Science, 26*(4), 960–979.

Bartel, C. A., & Garud, R. (2009). The role of narratives in sustaining organizational innovation. *Organization Science, 20*(1), 107–117.

Boje, D. M. (1991). The storytelling organization: A study of story performance in an office-supply firm. *Administrative Science Quarterly, 36*, 106–126.

Boje, D. M. (1995). Stories of the storytelling organization: A postmodern analysis of Disney as "Tamara-Land". *Academy of Management Journal, 38*(4), 997–1035.

Boje, D. M. (2001). *Narrative methods for organizational and communication research.* London: Sage.

Boje, D. M. (2008). *Storytelling organizations.* London: Sage.

Boje, D. M., Haley, U. C., & Saylors, R. (2016). Antenarratives of organizational change: The microstoria of Burger King's storytelling in space, time and strategic context. *Human Relations, 69*(2), 391–418.

Brooks, P. (1992). *Reading for the plot: Design and intention in narrative.* Cambridge, MA: Harvard University Press.

Brown, A. D., Gabriel, Y., & Gherardi, S. (2009). Storytelling and change: An unfolding story. *Organization, 16*(3), 323–333.

Bruner, J. S. (1990). *Acts of meaning.* Cambridge, MA: Harvard University Press.

Cunliffe, A., & Coupland, C. (2012). From hero to villain to hero: Making experience sensible through embodied narrative sensemaking. *Human Relations, 65*(1), 63–88.

Currie, G., & Brown, A. D. (2003). A narratological approach to understanding processes of organizing in a UK hospital. *Human Relations, 56*(5), 563–586.

Czarniawska, B. (2004). *Narratives in social science research.* London: Sage.

Dailey, S. L., & Browning, L. (2014). Retelling stories in organizations: Understanding the functions of narrative repetition. *Academy of Management Review, 39*(1), 22–43.

Downing, S. J. (1997). Learning the plot: Emotional momentum in search of dramatic logic. *Management Learning, 28*(1), 27–44.

Feldman, M. S., Sköldberg, K., Brown, R. N., & Horner, D. (2004). Making sense of stories: A rhetorical approach to narrative analysis. *Journal of Public Administration Research and Theory, 14*(2), 147–170.

Frandsen, S., Kuhn, T., & Lundholt, M. W. (Eds.). (2016). *Counter-narratives and organization*. Abingdon, UK: Routledge.

Fronda, Y., & Moriceau, J. L. (2008). I am not your hero: Change management and culture shocks in a public sector corporation. *Journal of Organizational Change Management, 21*(5), 589–609.

Frye, N. (1957). *Anatomy of criticism*. Princeton, NJ: Princeton University Press.

Gabriel, Y. (1995). The unmanaged organization: Stories, fantasies and subjectivity. *Organization Studies, 16*(3), 477–501.

Gabriel, Y. (2000). *Storytelling in organizations: Facts, fictions, and fantasies*. Oxford, UK: Oxford University Press.

Garud, R., Dunbar, R. L., & Bartel, C. A. (2011). Dealing with unusual experiences: A narrative perspective on organizational learning. *Organization Science, 22*(3), 587–601.

Georges, R. A., & Jones, M. O. (1980). *People studying people: The human element in fieldwork*. Berkeley, CA: University of California Press.

Gubrium, J. F., & Holstein, J. A. (1998). Narrative practice and the coherence of personal stories. *Sociological Quarterly, 39*(1), 163–187.

Humle, D. M., & Pedersen, A. R. (2014). Fragmented work stories: Developing an antenarrative approach by discontinuity, tensions and editing. *Management Learning, 37*(8), 1101–1124.

Lockett, A., Currie, G., Finn, R., Martin, G., & Waring, J. (2014). The influence of social position on sensemaking about organizational change. *Academy of Management Journal, 57*(4), 1102–1129.

MacIntyre, A. C. (1988). *Whose justice? Which rationality?* London: Duckworth.

Maitlis, S., & Christianson, M. (2014). Sensemaking in organizations: Taking stock and moving forward. *Academy of Management Annals, 8*(1), 57–125.

Martin, J., & Siehl, C. (1983). Organizational culture and counterculture: An uneasy symbiosis. *Organizational Dynamics, 12*(2), 52–64.

Mishler, E. G. (2004). *Storylines*. Cambridge, MA: Harvard University Press.

Pedersen, A. R. (2009). Moving away from chronological time: Introducing the shadows of time and chronotopes as new understandings of narrative time. *Organization, 16*(3), 389–406.

Pedersen, A. R., & Johansen, M. B. (2012). Strategic and everyday innovative narratives: Translating ideas into everyday life in organizations. *The Innovation Journal: The Public Sector Innovation Journal, 17*(1), 2–18.

Polkinghorne, D. E. (1988). *Narrative knowing and the human sciences*. Albany, NY: State University of New York Press.

Reissner, S. C. (2011). Patterns of stories of organisational change. *Journal of Organizational Change Management, 24*(5), 593–609.

Rhodes, C., & Brown, A. D. (2005). Narrative, organizations and research. *International Journal of Management Reviews, 7*(3), 167–188.

Rhodes, C., Pullen, A., & Clegg, S. R. (2010). 'If I should fall from grace. . . ': Stories of change and organizational ethics. *Journal of Business Ethics*, *91*(4), 535–551.

Sköldberg, K. (1994). Tales of change: Public administration reform and narrative mode. *Organization Science*, *5*(2), 219–238.

Sonenshein, S. (2010). We're changing - Or are we? Untangling the role of progressive, regressive, and stability narratives during strategic change implementation. *Academy of Management Journal*, *53*(3), 477–512.

Tsoukas, H. (2005). Afterword: Why language matters in the analysis of organizational change. *Journal of Organizational Change Management*, *18*(1), 96–104.

Vaara, E. (2002). On the discursive construction of success/failure in narratives of post-merger integration. *Organization Studies*, *23*(2), 211–248.

Vaara, E., & Pedersen, A. R. (2013). Strategy and chronotopes: A Bakhtinian perspective on the construction of strategy narratives. *M@n@gement*, *16*(5), 593–604.

Vaara, E., Sonenshein, S., & Boje, D. (2016). Narratives as sources of stability and change in organizations: Approaches and directions for future research. *Academy of Management Annals*, *10*(1), 495–560.

Van Maanen, J. (1988). *Tales of the field: On writing ethnography*. Chicago, IL: University of Chicago Press.

Weick, K. E. (1995). *Sensemaking in organizations*. London: Sage.

3 Making Sense of Everyday Innovation at a Clinical Ward Through Narratives of Visitation Routines

Is everyday life in a clinical hospital ward always the same? The answer is no. As stated in the introduction, health care organizations reflect the surrounding societies; therefore, routines in health care organizations are also continuously changing. Does change come from larger health care reforms, strategies, or radical innovations? Sometimes. But most of the time health care change can be understood as continuous change processes in clinical wards or other local units. These local change processes are a long way from political and top executives' strategy papers and reports. They happen almost as invisible change processes in the everyday routines and are not always visible for patients and external surroundings, but they are very real and time-consuming for the people working at the local wards.

The purpose of this chapter is to demonstrate how participants make sense and form narratives of a change process in a hospital ward. The first part of the chapter presents the theme of organizational change as a classical theme in organizational studies. The literature is divided into studies of episodic and continuous change (Weick & Quinn, 1999). A narrative approach of change processes implies an understanding of change as continuous, and as stated in Chapter 2, a narrative approach to organizational change consists of an understanding of the participants' sensemaking of change intentions and events, viewing change processes as intertwined with sensemaking processes. As organizational change in an everyday context involves change of routines, the literature on routines is presented to unfold how routines can be understood as not only tacit and unconscious repeated activities but also as dynamic, situated negotiations.

The second part of the chapter presents the empirical findings from an ethnographic study of an everyday change process in an emergency ward at a county hospital. The patients coming to the emergency ward arrive by ambulance, are referred from their general practitioner, or come in on their own initiative. The study followed the implementation of a new triage model to prioritize incoming patients. The study follows the introduction of a new triage model, a new way of prioritizing incoming patients through standardized steps leading to different color codes. The implementation of the visitation routine involved work standardization by assigning the incoming patients the colors green, yellow, orange, or red, reflecting their need for assessment. The emergency ward employed nurses, secretaries, and a few emergency chief doctors, but the majority of the doctors working in the ward came from other units in the hospital and had shifts in the emergency ward as a part of their overall schedule. The new routine involved nurses, incoming ward doctors, and the clinical manager, as well as patients (indirectly), as they did not know about the color codes but were waiting at the emergency ward to enter the hospital services.

The second part of the chapter presents the structured and fragmented individual narratives about the changing visitation processes. The structured narratives were told by the clinical manager to persuade health care professionals to follow the idea and the good intentions of the new visitation routine and by a patient who experienced the visitation from her illness perspective. The fragmented ante-narratives were told by the local health care professionals, both as counter-narratives, to resist the change process, and as more fragmented ante-narratives, to explain the unseen consequences of the new ways of organizing.

The contribution of the chapter is to demonstrate how these different individual narratives provide a picture of the polyphonic sensemaking conditions of everyday change and organizing.

Theories of Organizational Change as Everyday Innovation

Organizational change is explained in the organizational theory literature by two different theoretical strands: as episodic change and as continuous change processes. The understanding of organizational change in a health care setting is presented in this book from a continuous organizational change perspective. This means that change processes become part of everyday organizing. For a continuous change perspective to be applied to understand intentional local change projects, the concept of everyday innovation is presented as intentional local change projects within ongoing ways of organizing by redirecting sensemaking of local routines. As mentioned in Chapter 2, narrative frameworks are useful when a researcher is interested in how local participants make sense of change processes. This means that a change of routines needs to be translated into a local context, wherein organizational members and other participants make sense of these ideas in relation to their involvement in already established and negotiated routines.

From an Episodic Change to a Continuous Change Approach

An episodic change approach is based upon the understanding of effective change as planned and rational. This approach is in line with Lewin (1947), a social psychologist who developed his theoretical contribution on change as a three-step process, including: unfreezing the static organization, creating change, and refreezing the organization into a new, sound organization. Change should be initiated top-down by management, and Lewin proposed that managers should be particularly focused on planning and interventions in social groups as a means to create change. Lewin's ideas remain central to episodic change because they assume that inertia in the form of a quasi-stationary equilibrium is the main impediment to change (Schein, 1996 as cited in Weick & Quinn, 1999, p. 372). As it is natural to expect resistance to change, managers should identify important gatekeepers in the service production process. More recent studies promote the ideal that organizational change should derive from a top-down managerial orientation with a clear strategic vision (Fernandez & Rainey, 2006; Kotter, 1999/2012). Change concepts in the episodic change tradition include burning platforms, strategic change plans and visions, external and internal support, and change agents as effective prime movers. This change notion has become widely accepted as the main understanding change in health care change projects that are arranged from the top down (Fernandez & Rainey, 2006).

Weick and Quinn (1999) criticized the understanding of episodic change by presenting findings showing that most people who react in the action stage relapse and change back to previous habits three or four times before they maintain new sequences. This suggests that change is not a linear movement but rather a spiral pattern and process of contemplation, action, and relapses. They also underlined that to become a real change agent actors have to work on interpreting the actions of others, not as technical incompetence but as behaviors that are consistent with a particular cultural purpose, meaning, and history (p. 374). In contrast to episodic change, continuous change is based on the understanding that change is a neverending organizing processes. The concept of a loosely coupled system describes how change happens via appropriate actions and interactions in organizations (Weick, 1993). Weick suggested that respectful interaction depends on the presence of intersubjectivity, which provides an exchange and synthesis of meaning between two or more communicative selves and transforms the self in the interactive process in a way that adds to the development of a shared subjectivity. The assumption is that the change is driven by alertness and the ability of organizations to remain stable. The analytical framework specifies that contingencies, breakdowns, opportunities, and context make a difference, where change is an ongoing mixture of reactive and proactive modifications and redirections guided by the purpose at hand rather than an intermittent interruption of periods of convergence (Weick & Quinn, 1999, p. 379). In an episodic change approach, organizations are viewed as difficult to change, and change happens via strategic plans and designs. In a continuous change approach, change processes are viewed as constantly happening in organizations through ongoing change processes, wherein change processes happen through improvisation, translation, learning, and sensemaking (Weick & Quinn, 1999, p. 375).

There is one main consequence of applying a continuous change perspective in studies of organizational change. Recent studies of ongoing organizing processes (Hernes, 2014) pointed to how organizing is a processual, social process, and therefore is combined with ongoing sensemaking and narratives. One consequence of a processual organizational perspective is that change is not understood as deviant organizational behavior; instead, change processes, or constant movement, become the normal accepted condition of organizing. Accordingly, recent studies of organizing do not mention the words "organizational change," as change processes become an obvious part of the ongoing continuous processes of organizing. In this sense, the word "change" is no longer important to mention in studies of ongoing organizing processes. As a result, recent process studies no longer address change as a specific phenomenon that is different from ongoing organizing. Instead, everyday innovation addresses intentional, local change processes as part of continuous change processes that target changing local routines, which requires negotiation and sensemaking.

The Everyday as Negotiated Routines

What does the notion of the everyday mean? A repeated tacit activity in organizations? Research has explored the notion of everyday life in organizations, ranging from sociological studies (de Certeau, 1984; Deetz, 1992; Geertz, 1957; Goffman, 1959; Van Maanen, 1979) to more contemporary organizational studies (Denzin, 2003; Feldman & Pentland, 2003; Orlikowski, 2007; Ybema, Yanow, Wels, & Kamsteeg, 2013). These studies share a common interest in using everyday life as the object of study, often combined with the use of ethnographic methods. Goffman's (1959) classic studies of everyday life in a psychiatric institution entailed descriptions of two worlds split between the patients and the staff, with many everyday routines forming the identities of the patients. Goffman described how taking baths, dressing, and doing other daily activities demonstrated the dramas, tales, and institutionalization of everyday life.

De Certeau's (1984) book, *The Practice of Everyday Life*, outlines everyday life by describing the relationship between strategies and tactics. De Certeau described everyday life as a process of poaching on the territory of others, using the rules and products that already exist in the culture but seldom in the way the rules were intended. In other words, de Certeau made a distinction between territories (spaces) and strategies, defining everyday life as something other than rules, intentions, and strategies. He used the images of the layout of a city to explain that walking around a city never occurs as intended by city planners. Everyday life is then connected to "the road of daily living" and to the capacity to understand this perspective in contrast to strategy and plan making (Certeau, 1984).

These two classical everyday studies point to how descriptions of daily activities are a part of understanding everyday life and also how everyday life is a different territory compared to rules and strategies because a living condition in everyday life means that everyday life never turns out the way it was planned.

While it is difficult to describe uniformly all contemporary organizational studies of everyday life, they do share the common aim of looking beneath the surface of what appears to be something banal to explore the dilemmas, struggles, and complexities of everyday life. Bjørkeng, Clegg, and Pitsis (2009) concluded that most everyday studies define the everyday as embodied arrays of activities organized around a shared practical understanding of a "way of doing" under specific material configurations as kinds of social orders and particular practices (p. 146). As a result, everyday life studies examine the specific contextual condition of everyday life in many different organizational settings, ranging from haute cuisine (Gomez, Bouty, & Drucker-Godard, 2003; Svejenova, Mazza, & Planellas, 2007) to professional behavior in a law firm (Sandberg & Pinnington, 2009). Some of these contemporary studies of everyday life argue that everyday life is not about shared understandings, repetitive actions, and endless routines; instead, it involves a great deal of informal interactions, work, materiality, and complexity (Fayard & Weeks, 2007; Feldman & Pentland, 2003; Orlikowski, 2007; Ybema et al., 2013). Feldman (2000) defined how organizational routines are a source of continuous change, as they contain an internal dynamic through the inclusion of their participants. She argued that we need to relate routines to the people performing them and that change occurs as a result of participants' reflections and reactions to various outcomes of previous iterations of the routine (p. 611). Feldman and Pentland (2003) described how organizational routines have performative effects and how they can be changed if they are defined as internal dynamics instead of as inert structures wherein active agents work to change the routines. In accordance with Feldman's definition of organizational routines, organizational members can be understood as active participants of everyday routines that they negotiate and make sense of. In Feldman's later work (Pentland, Feldman, Becker, & Liu, 2012), organizational routines are defined by a generative model of action through the micro-foundation of routines as the things that actors do (p. 1484). Actors or people talk, both by doing or performing routines, but they also talk before and after by making sense of the routines. Routines are viewed as activities or events linked to interpretations and narratives as people make sense of their daily activities and negotiate their plans and ideas with their activities.

Thereby, organizational routines are situated in a context. This means that the situational or contextual local setting becomes important to understanding changing routines. Dopson, Fitzgerald, and Ferlie (2008) suggested that context should not be defined as a passive concept but

as an active, interacting component in the process of change and innovation: "It is not a backcloth to action; instead, local health care staff
engage in work practices and actively interpret and reconstruct its local
validity and usefulness" (p. 228).

Contemporary studies of everyday life stress how routines are not banal,
repeated activities but instead performative phenomena that are negotiated and context sensitive. Thus everyday life can be defined as dynamic,
negotiated routines. One good way to explore these dynamic routines is
through an everyday ethnography, as it makes it possible to follow and
describe in detail how sensemaking does not always result in shared understandings of these routines but also how different kinds of participation,
negotiation, and narrative create multiple sensemaking conditions.

Making Sense of Routines Through Narratives

One way of understanding everyday innovation is by investigating the
introduction of new routines and describing how local participants negotiate their ideas and their activities. One way of understanding their
dynamic interactions and negotiations is by listening to their narratives,
how they present new ideas, and how they negotiate the implementation
of these ideas into already existing routines. Pedersen and Johansen (2012)
emphasized the need to include different types of narratives, from managers' strategic spokesperson narratives to employee counter-narratives,
which allows participants in local change processes to express positive
and negative feelings toward the implementation of new routines.

Strategic spokesperson narratives are structured. Akrich, Callon, Latour,
and Monaghan (2002) described how trust defines our relations with others
and how spokespersons must be a legitimate and trustful presenters of the
idea (p. 219). The spokesperson formulates the strategies designed to persuade others to see the idea's good intentions. Strategic spokesperson narratives are thus important to creating coherence and a sense of new ideas and
to trying to persuade others by following the good intentions of the idea.

Everyday ante-narratives are unstructured and typically told by the
many voices of the employees, translating the idea into already existing
routines. These ante-narratives capture many different voices surrounding the innovation idea, stressing positive and negative elements in the
sensemaking processes (Hazen, 1994; Boje, 2008). Such ante-narratives
describe everyday innovation as fragmented, situational, conflicting, and
with unintended consequences.

Strategic spokesperson narratives and ante-narratives are related to
each other, as the former requires an audience to persuade. To become
public or outspoken ante-narratives, they need to be legitimized by the
management. The previously mentioned studies point to the importance
of unfolding both types of narratives in the everyday innovation process,
as the different narratives create very different sensemaking conditions.

Everyday innovation need not only include internal organizational members in studies of stability and change (Feldman, 2000; Pedersen & Johansen, 2012; Pentland et al., 2012) as including other participants can also be relevant. More concretely, patients are important stakeholders in a hospital context, who cannot be described as members of organizational routines but nonetheless play a part in participating in the routines. Studies of medical discourse have examined patient worlds as an important counterpart to medical and clinical studies (Kjær, Pedersen, & Pors, 2016). This field of research often problematizes the clinical encounter by pointing at the different aspects of patient versus medical narratives (Bury, 2001; Charon, 2005; Kelly & Dickinson, 1997). These studies demonstrate how illness narratives reveal patient perceptions and articulate how the patient experiences with illnesses can contrast with health care professionals' narratives and medical discourse (Apker, 2011; Bury, 2001; Charon, 2005; Kelly & Dickinson, 1997). Other studies have demonstrated how patient narratives created new insights into the patient experience by demonstrating voices from the worlds of patients in relation to the logic of health care professionals (Reay & Hinings, 2009; Pedersen, 2016). In other organizations, other external stakeholders would be relevant to include as participants in routines. In sum, as part of understanding everyday innovation, all kinds of possible participants in routines should be included, not only the organizational members, as they are often key participants in that they experience the routines and the history of the routines (Pentland et al., 2012).

Partial Discussion and Conclusion

The first section of this chapter presented two theoretical approaches to organizational change: episodic and continuous change. In a continuous change perspective, the notion of change is intertwined with the notion of organizing. This means that the study of organizational change also becomes the study of organizing. The notion of everyday innovation can instead explain intentional change processes of routines. Routines can be seen as dynamic, wherein the participants negotiate daily activities involving sensemaking and narratives. Strategic spokesperson narratives, as well as everyday ante-narratives, can be part of negotiating and making sense of new routines.

Overall, the theoretical part pointed to the difficulties of analyzing organizational change processes without also analyzing ongoing processes of organizing. In doing everyday ethnography, it becomes possible to study all of the small negotiations of how new ideas to change local routines (as with everyday innovation) require spokesperson narratives and also allow for narratives of all the unseen consequences of introducing a new way of organizing.

Spokespersons, Counter- and Patient Narratives About
Visitation Routines

The second part of this chapter presents a main sensemaking condition for organizational change in the form of different individual narratives. The analysis demonstrates the multiple and varied understandings of the daily routine of visiting incoming patients of a clinical manager, health care professionals, and a patient.

The three narratives are from an ethnographic study conducted at an emergency ward in a regional hospital. The study followed the implementation of a new triage routine at the ward, which can be described by the following daily events: after a patient arrives at the emergency ward and is registered by the secretary, and a nurse does an initial triage assessment of the patient's needs. This included, e.g., taking the patient's temperature, blood pressure, oxygen saturation, pulse, respiratory rate, and Glasgow Coma Score, as well as relating patient symptoms to a pre-defined emergency symptoms and signs algorithm. Then the values and symptoms are each designated a color code (green, yellow, orange, or red) applicable to the patient's assessment. This code is then registered on the patient's observation chart and given to the coordination nurse, who then lists the patients on a whiteboard. Upon registration, each patient is assigned a room number, which is recorded on the whiteboard, as well as the time of arrival, the patient's name, cause for contact, and which nurse is assigned to the patient.

The narratives were collected using the narrative framework presented in Chapter 2, including structured and fragmented individual narratives and the more specific narratives types presented in the last part of the theoretical section of this chapter: strategic spokesperson narratives, everyday ante-narratives, and patient narratives. The first narrative is by the clinical manager, who had the idea of making a new triage routine at the ward and acted as the spokesperson of the new idea. He had trained a nurse and was talking about his good idea and how he was working on translating it into everyday activities. He was a middle manager on the ward, serving as a liaison between its health care professionals and the head doctors and head nurse.

The second set of narratives examined are two ante-narratives told by participants, and they are fragmented, describing why it was difficult to translate and implement the triage ideas into the visitation routines. They talked about how changing the routines also brought unforeseen consequences for everyday innovation. Hence, these ante-narratives were both counter-narratives expressing resistance and fragmented ante-narratives expressing ambiguity and work frustration.

The last narrative is from a patient who had waited in the observation ward for several hours after arriving at the emergency ward. She was in a public waiting room, allowing her to follow the activities that occurred, her narrative reflecting her vantage point and her individual experience of being enrolled in the visitation routine on the ward.

These narratives were not chosen to express representative narratives told in the process; instead, they were chosen to represent the variety of narratives, demonstrating how a collection of local narratives of organizational change processes always entails multiple narratives and implying a fragmented sensemaking condition of the change idea and activities. The aim of this analysis is to demonstrate how the individuals participating in the routines tell narratives based on different everyday contexts and experiences; some wait in hallways or beds, others work in back offices, and others negotiate decisions by talking with others and walking through different areas.

The Clinical Manager's Strategic Spokesperson Narrative

In the following quote, the clinical manager who had the idea of implementing a new triage routine at the ward talks about why the triage model is an important way to work.[1] He talks about how the idea of using the triage model at the ward emerged from a need to change because the whole hospital area was changing. The project group he was a part of could see that the emergency ward would have more patients in the future and wanted to make patient pathways to care more efficient:

> A new hospital plan arrived, and we could see we would get more patients in the future, so we visited several places. We went to Beth Israel in Boston and Karolinska in Stockholm, and around in Demark. We spent six months, 2–3 people, and translated a Swedish triage manual from Swedish to Danish and included recommendations from the medical associations.
>
> (Clinical manager)

He mentions how a Swedish model inspired them and how they translated the manual from a Swedish cultural context into a national one by including professional values and advice from the national medical associations. The medical association provided important legitimation but was not the only stakeholder to do so. Support from the management team of the ward has also been crucial for him:

> It [support from the management team] has been undaunted and focused, and nothing has been said by the management team without it reflecting some kind of agreement. It was a completely formal deal/ agreement, also outwardly, that the management team backed up my strategy. And I didn't just make decisions without their backing/ support.
>
> (Clinical manager)

He relates to how trust from both the medical associate and the top management was part of making the decision to translate the Swedish visitation model into the local ward context. He then became the local spokesperson for the new triage model. Almost all of the health care professionals interviewed talked about the major role the clinical manager played in the change process. One nurse stated, for example:

> Who was the pioneer? It was [name of the clinical manager], no doubt about that. I've also worked under him as a nurse and already then he had these visions, visions of wanting to introduce triage in our emergency ward.

This shows that the clinical manager had the trust and support of the health care professionals, the medical associations, and the top management to translate the manual and activities into a local organizational context. He went around in the ward talking about why the triage idea was a good approach and would make improvements for the patients via safer and faster patient flow:

> If an elderly person comes in who fell on the street and got a hip fracture and she doesn't have heart or mental problems, then you can implement a very impressive process. We can make an optimized flow, where many patient flows look alike, and then we can be more prepared. . . . So, it's easier for us to standardize these processes in the hospital and also make room and space for more complex patients.
> (Clinical manager)

He thus explained why the new way of doing visitations was an improvement on earlier processes in which a good deal of time was used to perform tests and wait for test results and treatment plans. The clinical manager also had an explanation as to why the triage model was a better way of organizing the work in the ward than earlier practices:

> Earlier, I would spend a lot of time telling the doctor about all of the test results, but now the test results are in categories, so the patient gets a color, so the doctor automatically knows what the vitals are, when, say, it's a green patient. We can talk more about why the patient is here, which means the standardization model can speed the process up, and we can communicate in a safer way.
> (Clinical manager)

The clinical manager talked about the triage process presenting a standardization of the visitation work that can make the process of emergency visitation more effective and the collaboration between nurse and doctor easier. However, implementing the model into the existing routines caused resistance among some health care professionals, as the new work task of using color codes was viewed as a standardized work tool that challenged personal autonomy and professional judgment:

> Health professionals think they can just look at patients to see if they're pale, sweaty, and breathing quickly. Which means we can just look at them and we don't have to measure them. They say, I've been a nurse here for 25 years. I can see if a patient has low blood pressure.
>
> (Clinical manager)

> You can't come here and tell me about what things are like, and it's a long implementation process. We're open 24 hours, seven days a week, so I have to see if we're making mistakes and need to be more evidence based so we can correct our mistakes. I came in one morning after a nightshift. When I left at 10:30 pm, the triage system was working perfectly. When I came in the next morning, not one patient was marked with a color. The entire nightshift had simply decided I was a fool.
>
> (Clinical manager)

In these two accounts, the clinical manager openly and honestly described the resistance and the challenges of implementing the model in night shifts as he understood and accepted the breakdowns and relapses in the change process. Anyway, he never stopped advocating, believing that the new triage routines would improve the visitation of patients by being more efficient and based on evidence. The plot in his narrative was coherent, always focusing on the noble achievement of introducing the triage idea.

Ante-Narratives of Health Care Professionals

The health care professionals in the ward who had to translate the good idea for the triage into everyday routines told different stories about the implementation process.[2] Many of the narratives were ante-narratives, i.e., fragmented, not structured by a plot. One type of ante-narrative dealt with ambiguity and contrasting feelings of linking the triage model to the good idea but at the same time despising its implementation. One nurse described her ambivalent feelings toward the triage model:

> I think the teaching has been good, also from a Swedish nurse who has worked with it [triage] in Sweden. But compared to how they described it, it hasn't at all become like that here. So, the intentions are awfully good but in practice it doesn't work.

This small ante-narrative is one example, of which we heard many that were similar, dealing with the controversies of sharing the idea but not loving its implementation. The following statement is another example of a typical ante-narrative filled with contradictions:

> I felt like I was being split apart; I liked participating and selling the idea because it was a really good one, but I also had a leg in the other camp as an ordinary nurse. My frustrations dealt with wondering how we would ever make it work when the key person's function didn't even work. . . . The first day the key function had to start [key person was to guide the others through the new process], none of the key people were at work.
>
> (Nurse)

Many of these ante-narratives of ambiguity included tensions between the triage as both a good idea and as a system that did not work. These ante-narratives illustrate how the nurses interpreted and translated the triage model by contradicting the ante-narratives and talking about the positive improvements, while simultaneously mentioning negative implications.

One other type of ante-narrative for the nurses working with the triage concerned ambiguity by observing how the new routine led to unintended work consequences. Previously, the selection of patients, the division of patients between the nurses and doctors, and the amount of time patients waited were private decisions not visible to fellow employees. After implementation of the triage system, the employees' decisions became visible to everyone. One nurse explained:

> It's a good tool to show that [name] needs some help because she actually has two orange patients. And it's also a good tool to show that the other nurse has three patients, so it looks as if she is busy. But, well, she has three *green* patients and she's actually finished, so she can take some more.

The ante-narratives describe how the practice of color coding had unintended consequences for changing the nurses' work relations and their ability to plan their own work. More social control emerged regarding the workload of the nurses. This is an example of an unintended consequence in relation to collaboration and workload but intended in relation to prioritizing patients according to the level of acuteness. As a result, the ante-narratives of unintended consequences play a significant role in understanding the new visitation routine. The triage routine represented a difficult change process that meant adjustments to more than just one aspect of the emergency ward's everyday organizing. Several types of organizing changed, thus requiring the creation of many narratives in the attempt to understand all of the changes taking place.

Another ante-narrative of unintended consequences that arose involved standardization in contrast to experience because a key feature of the triage system is that it standardizes certain practices. This purpose also led to the creation of unintended consequences, as this interview sequence shows:

Nurse: But it [workflow] has also been changed by the fact that you also take people's skill level into account.
Interviewer: How?
Nurse: If you expect an orange patient and you have some idea of why he is orange then, as coordinating nurse, you might not give that patient to the youngest or most newly appointed nurse. You can always reevaluate later, when he is actually stable; then it's all right. So, in that way, you take people's abilities into account.

This ante-narrative deals with the complexity of the prior system of visitation, in which experience was an important competence in selecting patients. The narrative describes how experienced nurses could still use their knowledge when they had many patients with the same classification, a context in which they could still rely on individual skills to prioritize among patients. The last example of an ante-narrative of unintended ways of organizing involved the nurses' new routine of interviewing patients about their problems in a public hallway:

I think it went wrong when there were a lot of patients. There's no discretion regarding the patients. We have to ask them everything while they're sitting right next to each other and I can't take it. There, the ethics are gone, and that's wrong. In addition, you can say, we didn't do that before. Then, we looked more at the patient and said, 'Does this patient look ill or is it okay for him to wait, and can this patient wait while we receive this other patient?'

(Nurse, interview)

This ante-narrative illustrates how part of the new routine became unethical because patients were forced to describe their problems in a hallway where everyone could hear what was being said. Several of the nurses described a clash between ethics, which are perceived as a core value in nursing, and other values, such as quick treatment and quality of care parameters. This was explained due to the lack of congruence between the physical surroundings in the ward and the reorganization of their work according to the triage model; the physical space was not optimally suited to the workflow prescribed by the idea.

Together, these ante-narratives illustrate some of the new tensions emerging after working with the new visitation routine: the tensions between standardization of work and professional experience, between efficiency and ethics, and between liking the idea and despising its implementation. The ante-narratives also demonstrate the unseen organizing consequences of having new triage boards and routines as the workload of the nurses became visible, introducing social control, which caused ambiguity in understanding the value of the new visitation routines.

An Illness Narrative From an Incoming Patient

What do patients say? They were the center of the routines, as they were the people who had to be examined and prioritized after arriving at the ward. The patients arriving by ambulance were, of course, taken directly to a patient room. Non-acute patients typically sat in the public waiting room before being called into triage, either in a patient room or in the hallway if no vacant rooms were available due to the quantity of patients. The following narrative is from the researcher's interviews and field notes and is about Mary (fictional name), who was interviewed during her stay in the observation room after waiting some while at the ward. She provides an example of a narrative from a patient waiting in the emergency ward:

> Mary explains that she went to her GP first when she felt sick, tired, and had no energy. The GP referred her to the hospital and had arranged for transportation since the doctor had found her incapable of driving on her own. She arrived at the hospital in the afternoon and was dropped off just outside the entrance. She then walked to the counter, where she was registered by a nurse and told to take a seat and wait to be called in. At dinner time, she had blood samples taken and, in the evening, she was told that the tests showed elevated values and that she had to wait for a doctor. When the doctor finally arrived, he told her that it was too late in the evening to do a scan, so he gave her an anticoagulant injection and told her to go home and come back the next day for an ultrasound. When Mary had asked about the waiting time, she was told that she was second on the list, but acute patients kept on arriving and had to be treated first. Mary stated, 'I felt like I waited forever, especially because I was concerned about my condition and not feeling well.' She adds, 'When you're on the emergency ward, you expect things to happen.' The time went slowly, which Mary emphasized by pointing out that the nurses started recognizing her when they passed her in the hallway and asked, 'Are you still sitting here?' Mary also talked about how she was sitting across from two rooms where patients came in and out, but that she did not see anyone tidying up or doing any cleaning during the many hours she waited just outside. Quite upset, she repeated that, despite the fact that several patients were treated in the room, no one did any cleaning for the entire eight hours she waited.

I asked her if she experienced other issues besides the long wait and she replied, 'Well, no, except for the fact that I was starving. There was water available and we finally got a cup of coffee, but no food.' Mary also talked about how she went to the office at one point to ask if she could go home, but was informed that they had to examine the blood test results first. When Mary was finally told that she could go home but had to come back the next day for further tests, it was almost midnight. She had hoped that she would find out was wrong so that she could look forward to the right treatment. Because it was so late, the free patient transportation service was no longer running, and she had to call and wake up her daughter to bring her home. In the end, Mary returned home shortly after midnight.

In the narrative Mary described the emergency ward as a place where time passes slowly. She thus represented the various patients who come in and out of the ward every day. Mary's narrative is special because it became a silent narrative, only told to the researcher or other patients, and was not a part of the formal visitation and medical conversations. Her narrative reflects the patient view on her stay and addressed the individual illness condition of understanding her situation as a patient in the emergency ward. She was part of the visitation routine, a routine she was not familiar with, but she related to it as she reflected on values such as cleaning, food, and transportation, which none of the organizational members were talking about. This patient narrative demonstrates another perspective on routines through the experience of participating in them without having influence on them.

Discussion and Conclusion

The clinical manager shared a structured and strategic spokesperson narrative of the good intentions of introducing the triage model at the ward. The plot of the narrative described victories, struggles, and recognition (we can optimize flow, we can correct our mistakes, etc.). Thus, this narrative develops like an epic narrative (Gabriel, 2000), which means it was also strategic, with the goal of persuading health care professionals to believe that triage created faster and safer treatment of patients, making it a good idea. This narrative is, in many ways, in direct conflict with the patient narrative. This was a structured tragic/comic narrative of undeserved misfortune (Mary talked about being number two in line but being overtaken by acute patients). She had to wait a long time, starving, feeling sorry for herself and fearful about not getting results (she talked about being concerned with her condition). These narratives demonstrate how difficult it is to establish a shared understanding of a good idea, as some will be the losers of the system, i.e., Mary did not experience rapid patient flows. So even though the new triage model selects patients in a more evidence-based way, not all patients will experience that as an improvement for their individual treatment and illness trajectories. Instead, patient values such as waiting time, hygiene, food, and transportation are emphasized. In this case, the patient narrative represented moral values related to client responsiveness, and the clinical manager represented moral values in relation to fairness (acuteness) and two democratic values related to street-level theories, explaining the relationship between front workers' engagement with clients/citizens (Zacka, 2017).

The health care professionals' ante-narratives illustrated how ambiguity and tensions were part of discussing and understanding how the triage idea was translated into a routine. A crucial aspect of ante-narratives is that they allow for uncovering contradictions and tensions, and here they created spaces for the nurses to generate critical opinions during the implementation of the triage idea. The ante-narratives illustrated many of the theoretical elements from the continuous change perspective, where relapses, breakdowns, and redirections were part of the change processes. They also demonstrated how change processes were intertwined with everyday organizing, as the new routines had many unseen organizing consequences: more visible workloads, social control, standardization of work tasks, and unethical conversations, which were never part of the arguments as to why the triage idea would improve the patient flow. Thus the example of how the triage idea was translated into new routines has demonstrated how organizational change processes make sense for health professionals and support strong engagement and, consequently, the role of the health care professionals in change processes, as the next chapter will further illustrate.

The three narratives described earlier share a condition, as they, in Goffman's (1959) terminology, are backstage narratives being told about work scenes in a waiting room and in offices for personnel only. Thus they represent the fragmented sensemaking condition of organizational change processes, and ethnographic studies make it possible to describe them. According to de Certeau (1984), they also represent different spaces or territories: patients in waiting areas and patient rooms a long way from busy health care professionals working on the triage board in assessment rooms to determine color codes. They are breaching the spaces or territories of others when they meet but seldom in the ways that they expected to. Together, these narratives show how change does not always happen from shared and collective sensemaking. Instead, new routines in everyday life in a clinical setting require sensemaking negotiations between clinical managers and health care professionals, and as an unseen result, patient narratives become the silent voices and represent how the patient perspective is not an integrated part of changing everyday organizing at hospital wards.

Finally, the narratives illustrate everyday innovation with the intention to change routines. Everyday innovation included patient reflections on their illness trajectory, the clinical manager's intentions of introducing evidence-based visitation routines, and health care professionals balancing the implementation of these routines with patient needs and work conditions. Hopefully these narratives provided a useful snapshot of the sensemaking conditions of everyday innovation at hospital wards by including various sensemaking conditions of how new visitation routines can result not only in active decision making and negotiations but also in slow and disappointing wait times.

Notes

1. Parts of these accounts are also presented in the following rapport: Johansen, M. B. (2010). Innovation og triagearbejde-en kvalitativ undersøgelse af triage på Akutafdelingen, Hillerød Hospital. *Center for Health Management, Copenhagen Business School, Copenhagen,* 1–66.
2. Parts of these accounts are also presented in the rapport: Johansen, M. B. (2010). Innovation og triagearbejde-en kvalitativ undersøgelse af triage på Akutafdelingen, Hillerød Hospital. *Center for Health Management, Copenhagen Business School, Copenhagen,* 1–66.

References

Akrich, M., Callon, M., Latour, B., & Monaghan, A. (2002). The key to success in innovation part II: The art of choosing good spokespersons. *International Journal of Innovation Management, 6*(2), 207–225.

Apker, J. (2011). *Communication in health organizations.* Cambridge, UK: Polity.

Bjørkeng, K., Clegg, S., & Pitsis, T. (2009). Becoming (a) practice. *Management Learning, 40*(2), 145–159.

Boje, D. M. (2008). *Storytelling organizations.* London: Sage.

Bury, M. (2001). Illness narratives: Fact or fiction? *Sociology of Health & Illness, 23*(3), 263–285.

Charon, R. (2005). Narrative medicine: Attention, representation, affiliation. *Narrative, 13*(3), 261–270.

de Certeau, M. (1984). *The practice of everyday life.* Berkeley, CA: University of California Press.

Deetz, S. (1992). *Democracy in an age of corporate colonization: Developments in communication and the politics of everyday life.* Albany, NY: State University of New York Press.

Denzin, N. K. (Ed.). (2003). *Performance ethnography: Critical pedagogy and the politics of culture.* London: Sage.

Dopson, S., Fitzgerald, L., & Ferlie, E. (2008). Understanding change and innovation in healthcare settings: Reconceptualizing the active role of context. *Journal of Change Management, 8*(3–4), 213–231.

Fayard, A. L., & Weeks, J. (2007). Photocopiers and water-coolers: The affordances of informal interaction. *Organization Studies, 28*(5), 605–634.

Feldman, M. S. (2000). Organizational routines as a source of continuous change. *Organization Science, 11*(6), 611–629.

Feldman, M. S., & Pentland, B. T. (2003). Reconceptualizing organizational routines as a source of flexibility and change. *Administrative Science Quarterly, 48*(1), 94–118.

Fernandez, S., & Rainey, H. G. (2006). Managing successful organizational change in the public sector. *Public Administration Review, 66*(2), 168–176.

Gabriel, Y. (2000). *Storytelling in organizations: Facts, fictions, and fantasies.* Oxford, UK: Oxford University Press.

Geertz, C. (1957). Ritual and social change: A Javanese example. *American Anthropologist, 59*(1), 32–54.

Goffman, E. (1959). *The presentation of self in everyday life.* Garden City, NY: Doubleday.

Gomez, M. L., Bouty, I., & Drucker-Godard, C. (2003). Developing knowing in practice: Behind the scenes of haute cuisine. In D. Nicolini (Ed.), *Knowing in organizations: A practice-based approach* (pp. 100–125). London: Taylor & Francis Group.

Hazen, M. A. (1994). Multiplicity and change in persons and organizations. *Journal of Change Organizational Management, 7*, 72–81.

Hernes, T. (2014). *A process theory of organization.* Oxford, UK: Oxford University Press.

Kelly, M. P., & Dickinson, H. (1997). The narrative self in autobiographical accounts of illness. *The Sociological Review, 45*(2), 254–278.

Kjær, P., Pedersen, A. R., & Pors, A. S. (2016). A discursive approach to organizational health communication. In E. Ferlie (Ed.), *Oxford handbook of health care management* (pp. 302–325). Oxford, UK: Oxford University Press.

Kotter, J. P. (2012). *Leading change.* Cambridge, MA: Harvard Business Press.

Lewin, K. (1947). Frontiers in group dynamics: Concept, method and reality in social science, social equilibria and social change. *Human Relations, 1*(1), 5–41.

Orlikowski, W. J. (2007). Sociomaterial practices: Exploring technology at work. *Organization Studies 28*(9), 1435–1448.

Pedersen, A. R. (2016). The role of patient narratives in healthcare innovation: Supporting translation and meaning making. *Journal of Health Organization and Management, 30*(2), 244–257.

Pedersen, A. R., & Johansen, M. B. (2012). Strategic and everyday innovative narratives: Translating ideas into everyday life in organizations. *The Innovation Journal: The Public Sector Innovation Journal, 17*(1), 2–18.

Pentland, B. T., Feldman, M. S., Becker, M. C., & Liu, P. (2012). Dynamics of organizational routines: A generative model. *Journal of Management Studies, 49*(8), 1484–1508.

Reay, T., & Hinings, C. R. (2009). Managing the rivalry of competing institutional logics. *Organization Studies, 30*(6), 629–652.

Sandberg, J., & Pinnington, A. H. (2009). Professional competence as ways of being: An existential ontological perspective. *Journal of Management Studies, 46*(7), 1138–1170.

Schein, E. H. (1996). Culture: The missing concept in organization studies. *Administrative Science Quarterly*, 229–240.

Svejenova, S., Mazza, C., & Planellas, M. (2007). Cooking up change in haute cuisine: Ferran Adrià as an institutional entrepreneur. *Journal of Organizational Behavior, 28*(5), 539–561.

Van Maanen, J. (1979). The fact of fiction in organizational ethnography. *Administrative Science Quarterly, 24*(4), 539–550.

Weick, K. E. (1993). Organizational redesign as improvisation. In G. P. Huber & W. H. Glick (Eds.), *Organizational change and redesign: Ideas and insights for improving performance* (pp. 346, 379). Oxford, UK: Oxford University Press.

Weick, K. E., & Quinn, R. E. (1999). Organizational change and development. *Annual Review of Psychology, 50*(1), 361–386.

Ybema, S., Yanow, D., Wels, H., & Kamsteeg, F. H. (Eds.). (2013). *Organizational ethnography: Studying the complexity of everyday life.* London: Sage.

Zacka, B. (2017). *When the state meets the street: Public service and moral agency.* Cambridge, MA: Harvard University Press.

4 A Resistance and Everyday View on Health Care Professionals

The purpose of this chapter is to demonstrate how resistance to everyday innovation and organizing can be explained through observation of interactions and identifying the local values of health care professionals. The main argument in this chapter is that to understand the role of health care professionals in everyday innovation, we have to investigate their local interactions in daily routines as well as identify their local values, as they will indicate whether the health care professionals would be inclined to participate in new change projects or be likely to resist.

The first part of the chapter presents classical theories of professions. Evetts (2003) stated that most analyses of professionalism as a normative value system have been at macro- and meso-levels of inquiry (p. 399). In contrast to this focus, everyday innovation and organizing are per se a micro-level exploration of health care professionals, with a focus on their meeting routines. Meetings are a type of a routine used to accomplish organizational work (Feldman, 2000, p. 611). Meetings in organizations also happen due to the need for organizing and the daily coordination of work (Schwartzman, 1989, p. 22). They can serve for negotiation, making decisions, hearing different perspectives, or clarity in communication. Weick (1979) described how meetings provide a sense of what that is going on for participants (p. 133). The professional-patient meeting is a particular type of meeting routine between the patient and, e.g., the doctor, during which professionals use their professional roles to interact with patients representing an illness/patient perspective (Kleinman, 1988). Multidisciplinary meetings, on the other hand, often reflect medical dominance (Kjær, Pedersen, & Pors, 2016; Mishler, 1984). Earlier studies have demonstrated the importance of health care professionals to organizational change processes (Fitzgerald & Ferlie, 2000). In some studies, health care professionals have been identified as the strongest opponents of organizational change because they represent strong profession-oriented values and logics and expect autonomy over work tasks, which can make change processes difficult (Sehested, 2002).

The second part of the chapter presents an organizational ethnography at a rehabilitation hospital. The hospital was responsible for the rehabilitation of patients following treatment in orthopedic, rheumatologic, medical, and neurological wards in other hospitals. The patients were often amputees, arthritis patients, and those coping with cerebral hemorrhage or injuries sustained in a fall. The health care professionals were nurses, physicians, assistant nurses, a social counselor and a large number of occupational therapists and physiotherapists. The study followed everyday organizing and innovation at the ward because a local change project was being introduced during the field work, with the aim to collect data from the entire nursing student population of the hospital at one ward. This project met with resistance from the health care professionals at the ward, who argued that it would take away valuable time spent with patients if they had to include the nursing students in their daily activities, in addition to medical encounters and multidisciplinary meetings.

In the second part of the chapter, two types of narratives are presented. The first narratives are about the clinical encounter, with professionals reflecting on their relations to patients and how these relations are part of forming their local professional values. The second analysis presents fragmented ante-narratives from multidisciplinary meetings, demonstrating how professions collaborate with one another through their understanding of each other as professional groups.

The narrative analysis includes individual structured narratives and more fragmented individual ante-narratives (as described in Chapter 2). This makes it possible to identify the strong values of health care professionals that are formulated in more structured narratives, whereas they talk about their values in regard to patient interactions and the struggles and tensions between different professional groups, which are told more as counter-narratives and ante-narratives.

The contribution of this chapter is to demonstrate how professional values and struggles in processes of everyday innovation at a clinic dominate sensemaking conditions.[1]

Theories of Health Care Professionals in Organizations

Sociological studies of professions in health care have illustrated many important topics examining the formation of the medical professions and the general processes of professionalism in health care. Concepts such as jurisdictions, control, power, autonomy, knowledge, authority, boundaries, legitimacy, and social roles and identities have all defined professions as a distinct occupational type in different ways. First, various fundamental concepts in the sociology of professions will be briefly presented. Then two strands of research will be presented, the development of professions as modern occupational groups in organizations, followed by a focus on their struggles over values and logics.

Professions as Groups With Autonomy and Knowledge

The formation of professions is a well-described field of knowledge, and theories of professions are a classical sociological discipline. Classical studies of professions have endeavored to understand the conditions under which a profession is cultivated in society (Abbott, 1988; Freidson, 1970; Parsons, 1939). Parsons (1939), often described as the founding father of the theory of professions, examined the similarities between professionals and business people and found that both applied scientific knowledge to address social needs, with the difference being that business people pursued self-interest, whereas professionals were culturally compelled to act altruistically and place welfare ahead of personal gains. Parsons understood professions as a common good for society because they serve the greater good instead of serving self-interest. He defined professions as possessing emotional neutrality and a symmetrical relation to citizens, and as being loyal toward their professional groups. In that sense, professions serve society, much like the public sector, in contrast to the business world's focus on self-interests.

Abbott's (1988) aimed to understand the formation of the professions, and he described how certain conditions were important to this process. His most well-known description is the areas of work over which certain occupational groups have control, which he labeled "jurisdictions." Through establishing jurisdictions and the understanding of the professions' ability to constitute a system, professions could define their workplace and culture, public opinion, and their legal and administrative rules. He described how professions battled over different jurisdictions because the strongest profession had a strong monopoly and a core jurisdiction, but nonetheless they operated as part of an interdependent system, with fluid boundaries between the jurisdictions.

Following these studies, a large number of more critical studies of professions emerged. Wilensky's famous 1964 article asked, "Do we experience the professionalization of everyone?" He argued that not all occupational groups could be characterized as professional. Freidson (1970) followed with a focus on the institutional contexts of the professions and the concept of occupational closure. Occupational closure defines how certain professional groups have a strong self-understanding, and they work on maintaining their status in society by erecting barriers and borders to protect their self-interest as powerful and important groups in society with strong degrees of autonomy and an interest in maintaining legitimate control over their work.

There have been many efforts to define the history of professions and their role in society (Burrage & Torstendahl, 1990; Dent & Whitehead,

2013; Larson, 1979; Mik-Meyer, 2017). Among other considerations, some studies explored the relations between the professional and the state, the power of professions, management versus professions, and the progression of professional identities. Often studies of professions are either critical toward professional groups and the effort to maintain power and dominance over other groups in society in self-interest, or they are more positive, describing the benefits of professions in society and their altruistic values. This division in the history of the theories of professions is combined in recent studies, demonstrating both the critical as well as the more valuable conditions of societies with large groups of professions. An example of topic in these studies is the question of how the cultural values and beliefs of professions are created throughout strategies, wherein they can ensure a monopoly of a work area and management control through collegiality and building internal trust relations (McNeil, Mitchell, & Parker, 2013).

Strong professional groups are often described as lawyers, priests, and engineers, as these roles represent individual agents with a large degree of specialized knowledge. Larson (1979) described that Anglo and continental understandings of the concept of professions have differed. The Anglo-oriented view of professions understands professionals as practitioners with a large degree of freedom to control their own workplace and a high degree of self-regulation. In contrast, the continental model of professions understands professions as elite administrators with academic credentials (Larson, 1979). Some of the first studies of professions in health care were on physicians and medicine (Bucher & Strauss, 1961; Freidson, 1970; Hunter, 1991; Larson, 1979; Mishler, 1984; Parsons, 1939). Physicians are often characterized as classic professionals with exclusive control over an abstract body of knowledge and autonomous practices (Freidson, 1988). In his study, Freidson observed how physicians achieved a position of professional dominance, allowing them to control the content of their own work, in addition to the work of fellow medical workers. Some studies of physicians examined how medical students are initiated into a system that is self-governing (Bucher & Strauss, 1961). Other studies related to professional control and power, wherein physicians have a monopolistic position, requiring authorizations and credentialing for specialized skills to maximize their status and control of other members of the medical professions (Larson, 1977).

The studies of professions in health care expanded, covering a broad rise in multiple health care professions, e.g., nurses, occupational therapists, midwives, caregivers, laboratory scientists and technicians, radiologic technologists, and medical assistants, all of whom are health care service providers within a system of professions (Abbott, 1988). Contemporary studies have looked at how boundaries between health care professionals are important to establishing and reproducing domains and how power dynamics across professional groups are a source for understanding change and resiliency in health care organizations (Fournier, 2000; Reay, Goodrick, & Hinings, 2016). New studies of the medical professions are finding new challenges for the professions: patient consumerism, the rise of evidence-based medicine, the increasing power of the pharmaceutical industry, and how resilience of the medical professions are a part of the transformation in response to these challenges (Timmermans & Oh, 2010).

Classical studies of professions stress the importance of autonomy, jurisdictions, and occupational closure and how new societal and cultural conditions affect their development, especially in relation to health care professionals. The new technological possibilities make them an even more important group, as they have the knowledge to prioritize between them.

Development of the Roles of Professions in Organizations

One theme in the literature of professions is the development of the new roles of the professions. Noordegraaf (2007) argued that Wilensky's famous question had not lost its relevance. Society today still faces pressures to professionalize all sorts of occupational domains, but the occupational control has moved to managerial control, with evidence-based and outcome-oriented movements blending in with professionalization efforts (p. 764). This means that the role of professions today is contested, and new roles are emerging, bringing hybridized images of professionalism, with new types of reflexive control to establish a meaningful connection between clients, work, and organized action. To describe this development Noordegraaf identified the different types of professional roles present today, representing an ongoing battle over the definition to determinate what a professional is (see Table 4.1).

Table 4.1 demonstrates two views on professions—the purified professions, describing the traditional professions that can be related to technical rationality, and knowledge-intensive occupational practices, which are highly specialized but still modifiable through self-regulation. This view on professionalism establishes occupational closure, such as to membership as well as professional identity. The pure professions are guided by highly educated skills, a service ethic, and a code of conduct that guides appropriate professional interaction and reaction (Noordegraaf, 2007, p. 766). The control system for purified professionalism is established by the professions themselves, and they are part of professional fields with boundaries closed from the outside world, based on moral conduct and normative and ethical control (p. 767). This view on professions is challenged when professionalism is related to ambiguous domains, wherein knowledge societies are contested, complex, unstable, and represent value conflicts. When competing guidelines and methods make objectification more difficult, knowledge becomes a contested field. When legitimacy is related to capacity problems and scarce resources, it becomes difficult to establish strong closed associations, and when networked societies call for flexibility, specialized knowledge and intuitional

Table 4.1 Types of Professional Roles

	Content /Substance (Knowledge, Ethics)	Institutional Control (Jurisdictions, Codes Of Conduct)
PURIFIED PROFESSIONS	Knowledge-intensive practices Codification of professional skills and education Act according to shared service ethic Reject the idea of professionalism outside of traditional professional domains	Supervisor for professional conduct Part of professional field with boundaries Professional control Professional knowledge should overrule managerial knowledge
SITUATED AND HYBRIDIZED PROFESSIONS	Contested knowledge domains Competing methods and guidelines Act according to capacity problems Links with the outside world are part of professionalism	Professional control is criticized Destabilized institutional power and shifting boundaries Institutional and network control Professions are reflexive practitioners in organizational contexts

Source of inspiration: Noordegraaf, 2007

power become destabilized and boundaries begin to shift. In this view, professions interact with organizational control, and professional and managerial roles become more blurred. This calls for a new definition of professions, so instead of defining professional work as a model of technical rationality, the professional work is related to the use of a reflexive practice in situations of uncertainty. Professions make sense of situations, relationships, roles, and objects by relying on knowledge that is taken for granted and through continuous interpretation, meaning construction (Noordegraaf, 2007, p. 774), and reflexive control. Noordegraaf concluded that this development has left us with a hybridized interpretation of professionalism, which has no definitive epistemological grounds but is about controlling the meaning of control itself. When control of meanings becomes a central element in understanding professions, one way to make sense is through narratives. There have been numerous narrative studies of health professions, illustrating how different professionals talk and shape their meanings and values through narratives (Bury, 2001; Hunter, 1991; Kleinman, 1988; Loewe, 1998).

The study of the development of the roles of professions highlights the fact that professions can enter different roles, and there are hybrid roles, which have to be negotiated and made sense of in a continuous battle of navigating to define what a professional is (McGivern, Currie, Ferlie, Fitzgerald, & Waring, 2015; Noordegraaf, 2015).

Struggles Over Values or Institutional Logics

Another recent theme in studies of professions is the understanding of their struggles. For many years, there has been a close connection between institutional theory and new understandings of professions. Health care systems are both highly institutionalized and highly professionalized (Borum & Westenholz, 1995). The assumption in many studies of processes of institutionalization in health care is that health care organizations respond to changes in their environment—not only to technical demands but also to normative and regulative forces (Alexander & D'Aunno, 1990; Reay et al., 2016; Scott, Ruef, Mendel, & Caronna, 2000). This means that health care systems' tendencies to reproduce the status quo, and the professionalized nature of health care, result in the traditionally conservation professions holding power to resist imposed change and maintain stability (Reay et al., 2016). Contemporary institutional studies have described how different types of institutional logics are present in health care, and how they sometimes represent competing power dynamics across professional groups via competing institutional logics (Reay et al., 2017). Table 4.2 is based on inspiration research by Reay and Hinings (2009) and their description of two rival, competing institutional logics in the health care field in Alberta, Canada.

Reay and Hinings's study demonstrated how competing logics and institutional change are tightly connected when institutional logics become the organizing principle because they challenge a set of belief systems and practices defined by meanings. When a new logic is introduced to an established field, rivalry among key logics is likely to happen as the newcomers are challenging the dominant logic (p. 632). These findings are supported by other studies of change in health care, such as Ferlie and Geraghty's (2005) study on public health care organizations that explored how professional culture can become a barrier to cross collaborative work and innovation, with resistance from the health care professionals. Also, Sehested (2002) stressed how public professions are under new pressures due to the new public management approach, leading to new roles in the professions as they are being controlled and managed more than ever before.

These studies stress the relationship between competing logics and change processes, as the institutional logics become organizing principles in contrast to preexisting sets of professional values or beliefs.

Partial Discussion and Conclusion

The theories of professions describe health care professionals as a distinct occupational group in society, with strong medical/health care values and strong belief in the value of self-regulation and autotomy in work

Table 4.2 Competing Institutional Logics

	Medical Professionalism	Business-Like Logic
VALUES AND LEGITIMACY	Save lives and heal with professional knowledge	Efficiency and doing more with less
AUTHORITY AND POWER	Autonomy and strong self-steering	Cost effective treatment; lowest cost
	Physicians are central to the delivery of quality health care and require appropriate resources to maintain position and autonomy	Physicians as cost problems Delivery based on evidence, citizen input, and government
	Principle: trust relations between patient and physician	Principle: accountability and government standards
PRACTICE PATIENT INTERACTION	Physician-patient relationship should guide all service provision	Customer satisfaction and advices and cooperation among all health care providers
	Physicians speak on behalf of patients	
ORGANIZING LOGIC	The role of government is to provide sufficient funds, as determined by physicians, which are the leaders of the health care system	The role of government is to provide efficient allocation of resources Physicians should carry out practices in accord with resource management guidelines

Source of inspiration: Reay & Hinings, 2009

tasks. The theories also leave us with an impression of a contested field, wherein professional logics struggle with more businesslike or managerial logics but also the jurisdictions between different health care groups remain contested and establish positions, boundaries, and power games, each being relevant topics to address.

When professions are defined as hybrid interpretations of professionalism, without a definitive epistemological ground, professionalism becomes about controlling meanings and narratives as a way to capture autonomy in the formation of meanings. The distinction between purified professions and situated professions can therefore be investigated by illustrating different types of narratives of knowledge domains, with contested or codified methods, skills, and practices.

Two themes demonstrating the contextual hybrid formation of the social roles of health care professionals and their struggles over values and logics were presented. These examples represent two central conditions of making sense of everyday innovation by including the perspective of professions.

Spending Time With Patients and Wasting Time in Meetings With Other Professions

The purpose of the second part of this chapter is to present an analysis of the micro-formation of values and struggles of health care professions, which are linked to possible resistance of changing everyday routines in a hospital ward. This study followed everyday organizing processes just before the nursing students arrived, to understand the profession's resistance against the project and how this resistance was bound to local routines: meeting patients and having meetings with other professional groups, as the health care professionals did not want to change these meetings with the inclusion of nursing students.

The analysis presents two types of narratives from health care professionals: individual, structured narratives about their encounters with patients, and individual, fragmented ante- and counter-narratives about their collaborations within the multidisciplinary meetings. The two types of narratives are from an ethnographic study conducted at a rehabilitation hospital. The study followed the everyday organizing at a ward, where everyday innovation continuously occurs. In particular, one example is provided of including all the hospital's nursing students in one ward. The local spokesperson of this project was a clinical manager, who told strategic spokesperson narratives of how collecting all of the nursing students into one ward would be a good idea, to enhance quality in learning and education.

In the rehabilitation hospital, the meetings with patients and other professions are very informal. In the ward, nurses and doctors work side by side with the patients in the patient rooms. The therapists and social counselors had separate locations at the hospital, so the patients went to therapy training sessions or to counseling outside of the clinic at other locations. The rehabilitation hospital had large training facilities. Physicians met with patients during the day but also nurses, therapists, and other professions, such as social counselors. This group then met to identify training problems and social/equipment issues experienced in the rehabilitation program. This multidisciplinary meeting was run on a weekly basis in this setting on every Wednesday at nine o'clock in the morning.

The first section presents two different narratives of how physiotherapist, Jane, and nurse, Eve, understand their interaction and values in patient interactions. Note that the narratives of patient encounters by nurses, therapists, and physicians differ, indicating that the professional educational background does not automatically represent a certain narrative (Pedersen, 2008).

The second part of the chapter presents a couple of ante-narratives and counter-narratives in the interpretations of collaborating with other professional groups at the weekly multidisciplinary meetings. The ante-narratives illustrate the difficult and competitive relationships between the various professional groups at the hospital.

The contribution of these analyses is to demonstrate how local values concerning patient encounters and local struggles between professional groups affect the sensemaking of local change processes. This explains why health care professionals in some cases resist change processes when they interfere with their local patient-related values and their internal struggles of defining their professional roles.

Jane's (Therapist) Narrative of Autonomy: Being Professional by Being Unprofessional

> If I were to characterize the good professional in a few words, it would be revealing to the patients who you are. I don't mind if the patients know where I live, how many children I have, and what I am doing in my leisure time. I find that sharing your life with the patients gives you a particular knowledge that may prove beneficial both to yourself as a professional and to the patient. This constitutes what some psychologists call a shared third. Sharing, for instance, my love of music with Mary means that when she's being discharged, I can tell her where and how she can attend concerts even though she is walking impaired. I have thus been able to help Mary with something that I think is of great importance to her, but which we would never have discussed had I not shared my interest in music with her. If I had only spoken with her about how to get dressed, cooking, shopping and such things that most physiotherapists discuss with their patients, I would never have learned about Mary's interest in music—it would never have emerged as a topic of discussion. However, others would probably call me rather unprofessional, especially when it comes to patients who I treat over longs periods. I share my thoughts and life with the patients, and I know that some of my colleagues find it a bad idea. But, for me, it's important to reveal who I am and to integrate the many aspects of my personality into the relationships that I am part of. I couldn't be physiotherapist Jane Petterson without telling my patients about myself. If I didn't, I would no longer find the job exciting.

Jane addressed her interaction with her patients and how she felt that informal talks and relationships were important for her to understand and connect with her patients. She reflected on her ability to have independent control (Freidson, 1988) over her work, which was not directed by others. Her professional choices highlighted the importance of sharing her thoughts with the patients. She interacted with patients, linking herself to outside worlds (Noordegraaf, 2007), which made her reflect on the relations between her professional position and her individual, personal ideas. The next story is from Eve, who is an experienced nurse.

Eva's (Nurse) Narrative of Knowledge: Being Professional by Being Experienced

> I regard the concrete meeting with the patient as closely tied to my experiences within the profession. Being a senior, experienced nurse who has encountered many different patients and their different problems over the years enables me to quickly recognize and define problems with new

patients. They remind me of something I've seen before, and I use my experiences actively when meeting new patients. Spending time with the patients and being attentive to their problems, no matter how big or small they are, is, for me, the core of being professional. Today, I involve myself much more than when I was younger, and over the years, I have become much better at advising and guiding patients. In my opinion, a good professional must have the courage to talk with patients about things that are inappropriate. For example, I find the economic situation between Mary and her husband highly unfortunate. I wouldn't be taking proper care of Mary if I neglected her remarks on the pretext of this being none of our business; she must decide herself if it is a private matter, etc. Medication, for instance, is a very sensitive issue, both among patients and among nursing staff, as patients react very differently to pain and to medicine. In my view, it's not enough, as a nurse, just to give the patients the medicine they are asking for. I wouldn't give in to Mary's request before having tried other solutions to alleviate pain. I let patients know that I feel sorry that they have back pain and that we must find a way of alleviating the pain, as more medicine will not help. In that way, I tell the patient, without giving in to her request for medicine, that I understand the request and her pain. This may result in [her feeling] stronger when she experiences that we can relieve her pain in ways other than by using medicine.

Eva presented herself as a pure professional (Noordegraaf, 2007), working with her knowledge and her professional skills to guide the patients. She reflected over her extensive work experience and how time had changed her view on being a professional. She noted the fact that she has to cover many care aspects, including difficult and simple issues. Both Eva and Jane share a strong feeling of ownership about caring for their patients and represent the needs and problems of their patients.

Together, these two narratives reflect the variety of understanding professional relations between professionals and patients—being professional meaning correct behavior in accordance with the values of the profession. The value of professional patient relationships ranges from distant to personal, demonstrating the autonomy professions have to interact with patients in different ways. The stories also reflect shared values, how their specialist knowledge about physical rehabilitation, care, and social problems became their core understanding of the patient's main problems. They all designate their relationship to the patients as the center of their attention, which reflects an Anglo-oriented understanding of professions (Larson, 1979) in which a large degree of freedom to control their own workspace and understanding themselves mainly as practitioners plays a central role. Interacting with patients is only a small part of the work life of professionals at the clinics. They also meet and talk with each other during their workday.

Becoming a Professional by Poaching on Each Other's Territories

Another type of organizing is the multidisciplinary meeting. In the rehabilitation hospital setting mono-disciplinary meetings were no longer
held. Instead, multidisciplinary meetings are places where they jointly
coordinate future activities and plans for the patients.

An observation from a multidisciplinary meeting describes examples of
the activities that take place during this type of meeting:

> The nurse takes the journal and places it prominently on the table,
> and then she says, "Then we have Mary." The physiotherapist speaks,
> sharing that Mary's memory has worsened. The occupational thera-
> pist interrupts and says that she does not have experience with that.
> The physiotherapist says okay, and that she will continue her team
> training with Mary, and that Mary has to learn to stop when it hurts
> because that is difficult for her. They others nod and say "Yeah." The
> occupational therapist shares that Mary was home over the weekend
> and that she had found her bloody clothes from the accident she was
> involved in, which was an unpleasant experience for her. The nurse
> breaks into the conversation. She also has told Mary that if she goes
> home on the weekend, it is important that she is not alone. "Well,"
> says the occupational therapist, "I just told her the opposite." "Can
> we just finish the memory part?" says the physiotherapist, "I have
> to continue as fast as possible." The occupational therapist explains
> why she disagrees about the memory issue and the group comes in
> with comments where they agree or disagree. "Okay," says the phys-
> iotherapist, "this is not going to change the things I will do with her,
> but it's nice, just to talk about her together." The physiotherapist
> leaves the room. The rest continue talking about Mary; they cannot
> agree on a common understanding of her, so they continue talking
> more quietly with their neighbors. In the end, they conclude some
> common decisions about Mary; the doctor then records them with
> her microphone (field notes from observation of weekly multidisci-
> plinary meeting at a rehabilitation ward).

This observation demonstrated the routines involved in discussing the
patient files by physically having the files on the table, where people sit
convened to discuss their different views of the patient's current conditions and treatment and conclude with jointly making future plans.

Ante-Narratives About Role Expectations

Talking with participants after a meeting resulted in multiple ante-
narratives about their view on their collaboration during the meeting,
their own expectations, and the others' participation:

Physiotherapist: I don't always think we manage to get each other aligned with the goals we're making for the patients at the meetings, we fall short in getting patient views included in the goals, but that's another story. We work based on the goals we have established, our shared goals, but I don't believe they are always shared, as not all professional groups speak up, and by that I mean the nursing group doesn't do that to a sufficient degree. The physiotherapist group thinks it's working on a shared goal, but it's not, but nobody disagreed when we discussed our thoughts.

Nurse: At the wards where I've been before the doctors always got the last word at the meetings and were extremely dominating, in contrast to other professional groups, but at this place, all groups are heard. Cross-disciplinary work, however, involves more than hearing from all of the professional groups; it involves being in a close dialogue, which doesn't yet exist at the meetings. It concerns the different options about the patients but also ownership: who owns the patients? If you ask the doctor, it's the doctor's patient, because he or she has the authority to prescribe medicine, writes in the medical file, possesses a broad overview, and can say yes or no. Do you ask the nurse if the patient is the nurse's patient, because she looks after the patient during the day and plays a motherly role? Do you ask the therapist, does the patient belong to the therapist because all of our patients undergo rehabilitation and training and that's the matter of concern? Maybe it's this way because we think too much about ownership and we all want to bring value to the patients but not in a shared dialogue.

Nurse: If I were to characterize the way we work now, I would say that work collaboration involves coordinating and making plans together at the meetings, but after these, there's no teamwork. Why can't patients go to the bathroom when they are training with the physiotherapist, but have to be taken down to the ward? Why can I, as a nurse, not train with the patients at the ward? Why is the therapist not at the ward during meals? Teamwork would involve nurses and therapists working together at the start of the day to plan the patients' day. Coworkers from other professional groups would be the close collaborative partners and all professional groups would be represented during the day and better integrated in the patients' lives than the current collaboration model.

These ante-narratives describe the difficulties involved in reaching shared goals, as each professional group has ownership of patients, and differing ideas they want to bring to the table. This makes it difficult to developing shared values or the shared third Jane mentioned. Instead, they talk about tensions between individual goals and shared goals and between hearing others and using this knowledge constructively.

These ante-narratives reflect a situated profession role wherein the nurses ponder the situated organizing and the competing methods (Noordegraaf, 2007). The ante-narratives demonstrate how situated professional values meet more purified professional values and show that the nurses reflect on how this clash makes meetings dysfunctional; as reaching shared goals becomes difficult each group has professionally defined patient ownership values as their start and end goals. These ante-narratives reflect some of the limitations of the medical professional logic (Reay & Hinings, 2009), where strong self-steering and professional speak-on-behalf-of-the-patient values create difficulties in creating teamwork and collaboration between the health care professionals.

Ante-Narratives of Struggling Professions

Some of the ante-narratives about the meetings were counter-narratives due to their highly critical stance toward the meeting format and the lack of professional boundaries established at meetings.

> Doctor: Sometimes there are remnants of old power games between physiotherapists and the nursing group, but that can be seen other places, too. In other words, the individuals who run these power games aren't concerned about the patients' different views; it's a proper power struggle concerning who is on the chart as a result of patient plans. Power struggles can occur at meetings when what the communication involves taking over to get your own opinion heard while suppressing that of others. Power games are frustrating and create an unsatisfactory working climate.
>
> Nurse: I get so frustrated about these meetings. The physiotherapists are so outspoken and talk about their opinions, while the nursing group, in contrast, is silent, all the while trying to get our act together to just say one or two things. I don't think we're good enough at putting ourselves out there and sharing our observations at the multidisciplinary meeting. The meetings shouldn't be postponed just because it's difficult for us to speak. Sometimes it feels like they just tell their information to the doctor and the fly out of door with excuses about waiting patients. Sometimes it feels like the physiotherapists aren't interested in our contact with the patients. I think they sometimes believe that, in comparison with their job, our work has the lowest status. . . . The professional boundaries become most visible at the meetings and less visible in the daily work. Even there, invisible boundaries exist that the nursing group can't cross to enter the physiotherapists area.
>
> Physiotherapist: I perceive the nurses as weak when it comes to meetings, and I don't think it has anything do to with their being used to the doctors being the ones who lead the discussion. This

weakness allows the therapists to be more controlling than we ought to be, and I think this makes collaboration difficult when we have to make joint decisions. That's a shame, since the nursing group, with their daily interaction with the patients, makes many excellent observations. At meetings, the nursing group lets me talk about the leg (after amputation), the training, prostheses, and various bandages, while other patient issues, such as relocation and taking a shower, have not been mentioned when discussing outpatients at meetings. My contact with the patients ends up being what we talk about at the meetings, even though the nurses, in most cases, have much more contact with them and know them better than I do.

These counter-narratives were told in opposition to the formal narrative, that health care professionals should work closely together and multidisciplinary meetings are an organizing event to support this idea. All of the participants talked about how these meetings include tensions between the professional groups and how a power game between the participants leaves some passive and others running out the door. The counter-narratives revealed how nurses are perceived as a weak professional group, and therapists are arrogant, directly telling the doctor what they think. The doctor talked about power struggle and how it relates to both professional groups and individuals, wherein it takes over and the doctor expresses an opinion by suppressing the views of others. These counter-narratives expressed the tensions and struggles between the various professional groups and individuals at the meeting; the meeting became a power arena, allowing dysfunctional patterns of communication without any single group being able to break them. Instead, the meeting was also a forum for competing logics (Reay & Hinings, 2009), wherein nursing and therapist logics were struggling as the hospital was not a traditional hospital dominated by physician logics (as described in one of the ante-narratives), allowing other competing health care logics to clash.

Discussions and Conclusion

The narratives demonstrated how spending time with patients is perhaps the strongest value in all of the professional groups and how spending time with each other perhaps became the weakest value for all of the professional groups in this study. This observation has major implications for understanding the possible resistance of professions to change processes. When a change project concerns values in relation to situated professional roles, such as having better coordination, planning, or quality in education, or in general, which requires more time spent in meetings, this leads to a natural rejection from some of the health care professionals, which was the case concerning changes in the nursing program.

Change processes that concern more time spent with patients have a better chance of being implemented, such as the triage change process in Chapter 3 because it makes sense to the health care professionals, as it aligns with their values of patient ownership (creating fairer patient trajectories). The new time spent with the patients reduced the autonomy of the professionals, as more work standards were introduced, but even the standards, as it turned out, required individual judgment (e.g., who can manage three orange patients).

The individual structured narratives used actions and emotions, such as exiting and feeling sorry, and described relations with patients. They also described interactions with the patient in detail, as well as the professionals' values related to these meetings (Pedersen, 2008). All of the narratives were epic, putting the professionals in the position of hero when helping patients. These narratives function as strong sensemaking devices for understanding their values in relation to their patients. Health care professionals, in a hospital context, can thus be characterized by having strong self-regulation in their daily patient encounters. The narratives of the professions at the rehabilitation hospital demonstrated how the value of the patient-professional relationship guided them and how the health care professionals speak on the behalf of patient needs.

The more individual fragmented ante-narratives also illustrated how the logic of medical professionalism (Reay & Hinings, 2009) was broken down into multiple micro-institutional logics, as the different professions, i.e., doctors, therapist, and nurses, talked about their own professional values being different and were in ongoing struggles with each other. These ante-narratives illustrated how ambiguity and tensions became part of understanding the meetings and the difficulties health care professionals had in working together at meetings. Meetings became a forum for power games, wherein implicit feelings of being a low status group became visible, resulting in silent participants.

But health care values and logics were also under development and continuous change, as purified, situated, and hybrid professional roles were in play (Noordegraaf, 2007). The meeting participants reflected about the contested knowledge domains and how competing methods caused limitations in collaboration. At the same time they explained their relationships with patients as an area of autonomy with professional control. This resulted not only in hybrid roles (McGivern et al., 2015) but also in reflections about the tensions and dilemmas between the purified professional values and situated professional values. Therefore, the rehabilitation health care professionals could be described as hybrid groups based on their reflections about competing methods and having purified values regarding patient ownership, with self-control or occupational closure making them distinct. But, in some cases they went beyond hybridization as organizing professionals as they reflected on the ongoing dilemmas of work as a mixture of organizational professionals, pure professionals, and coordinators because they were working in between competing log-ics and combining identities, but at the same time they represented pro-fessions and organizations that were responsible for coordination and organizing (Noordegraaf, 2015, p. 195).

This analysis does not present an understanding of the struggles between managers and professionals, or different values or institutional logics. The ward, which was driven by clinical managers, decoupled from the managerial layers of the hospital and the clinics, were mainly run with the participation of the health care professionals. Managerial tools ranging from new public management and other organizational business logics (Reay & Hinings, 2009) did not dominate the structuring routines and everyday organizing at the hospital. This means that this analysis mainly demonstrated the struggles and tensions among and between health care professionals as an ongoing sensemaking condition for orga-nizational change processes at the clinical hospital level.

The contribution of this narrative analysis is to unfold the strong and dominating, as well as the multiple and ambiguous, sensemaking condi-tions for health care professionals in everyday organizing. The counter-narratives about the meeting that were told to the researcher after the meeting, and the structured narratives told after having a personal medi-cal encounter with patients, were backstage narratives. They were told as part of an ethnographic study that allowed the researcher to be part of the daily activities, including observation and interviews, and were handled with a strong respect for openhearted storytelling. Such observa-tions and discussions allowed an outsider to get a picture of the blurred informal and formal conversations on hospital wards, as well as the sen-sitive aspects of forming a professional role when dealing with patients.

When trying to understand the ability of health care professionals to organize themselves in meetings and other daily organizing routines, the purified professional roles become barriers that the professionals must reflect upon. In other words, everyday innovations at hospitals are a con-dition of sensemaking of the patient relationship as a core professional value. This value can also make processes of innovation and coordina-tion beyond patient relationships difficult.

Note

1. The rehabilitation hospital is now closed as part of a restructuring wherein general therapy was moved from the regional hospital sector to local authori-ties, with specialized therapy being made available at the general hospitals. The analysis remains valid, as the same meeting routines currently still occur in all wards—that is, the clinical encounters between therapists/nurses/doc-tors and patients, as well as multidisciplinary meetings in which the health care professionals meet and discuss the patients' future treatment plans (with the patients' files physically on the table).

References

Abbott, A. (1988). *The system of professions: An essay on the division of expert labor*. Chicago, IL: University of Chicago Press.

Alexander, J. A., & D'Aunno, T. A. (1990). Transformation of institutional environments: Perspectives on the corporatization of US health care. In S. S. Mick (Ed.), *Innovations in health care delivery: Insights for organization theory* (pp. 53–85). San Francisco, CA: Jossey-Bass.

Borum, F., & Westenholz, A. (1995). The incorporation of multiple institutional models: Organizational field multiplicity and the role of actors. In W. R. Scott & S. Christensen (Eds.), *The Institutional Construction of Organizations* (pp. 113–131). London: Sage.

Bucher, R., & Strauss, A. (1961). Professions in process. *American Journal of Sociology, 66*(4), 325–334.

Burrage, M., & Torstendahl, R. (1990). *Professions in theory and history: Rethinking the study of the professions*. London: Sage.

Bury, M. (2001). Illness narratives: Fact or fiction? *Sociology of Health & Illness, 23*(3), 263–285.

Dent, M., & Whitehead, S. (Eds.). (2013). *Managing professional identities: Knowledge, performativities and the "new" professional* (Vol. 19). London: Routledge.

Evetts, J. (2003). The sociological analysis of professionalism: Occupational change in the modern world. *International Sociology, 18*(2), 395–415.

Feldman, M. S. (2000). Organizational routines as a source of continuous change. *Organization Science, 11*(6), 611–629.

Ferlie, E., & Geraghty, K. J. (2005). Professions in public service organizations. In E. Ferlie (Ed.), *Oxford handbook of health care management* (pp. 422–445). Oxford, UK: Oxford University Press.

Fitzgerald, L., & Ferlie, E. (2000). Professions: Back to the future? *Human Relations, 53*(5), 713–739.

Fournier, V. (2000). Boundary work and the (un)making of the professions. In N. Malin (Ed.), *Professionalism, boundaries and the workplace* (pp. 67–86). London: Routledge.

Freidson, E. (1970). Profession of medicine: A polemic. *Sociology of Health and Illness, 5*(2), 208–219.

Freidson, E. (1988). *Profession of medicine: A study of the sociology of applied knowledge*. Chicago, IL: University of Chicago Press.

Hunter, K. M. (1991). *Doctor's stories: The narrative structure of medical knowledge*. Princeton, NJ: Princeton University Press.

Kjær, P., Pedersen, A. R., & Pors, A. S. (2016). A discursive approach to organizational health communication. In E. Ferlie (Ed.), *Oxford handbook of health care management* (pp. 302–325). Oxford, UK: Oxford University Press.

Kleinman, A. (1988). Suffering, healing and the human condition. In R. Dulbecco (Ed.), *Encyclopedia of human biology* (Vol. 7, pp. 323–325). San Diego, CA: Academic Press.

Larson, M. S. (1979). Professionalism: Rise and fall. *International Journal of Health Services, 9*(4), 607–627.

Larson, M. S., & Larson, M. S. (1979). *The rise of professionalism: A sociological analysis* (Vol. 233). Berkeley, CA: University of California Press. Loewe, R.

(1998). Doctor talk and diabetes: Towards an analysis of the clinical construction of chronic illness. *Social Science of Medicine, 47*(9), 1267–1276.

McGivern, G., Currie, G., Ferlie, E., Fitzgerald, L., & Waring, J. (2015). Hybrid manager-professionals' identity work: The maintenance and hybridization of medical professionalism in managerial contexts. *Public Administration, 93*(2), 412–432.

McNeil, K. A., Mitchell, R. J., & Parker, V. (2013). Interprofessional practice and professional identity threat. *Health Sociology Review, 22*(3), 291–307.

Mik-Meyer, N. (2017). *The power of citizens and professions in welfare encounters: The influence of bureaucracy, market and psychology.* Oxford, UK: Oxford University Press.

Mishler, E. G. (1984). *The discourse of medicine: Dialectics of medical interviews* (Vol. 3). Westport, CT: Greenwood Publishing Group.

Noordegraaf, M. (2007). From "pure" to "hybrid" professionalism: Present-day professionalism in ambiguous public domains. *Administration & Society, 39*(6), 761–785.

Noordegraaf, M. (2015). Hybrid professionalism and beyond: (New) Forms of public professionalism in changing organizational and societal contexts. *Journal of Professions and Organization, 2*(2), 187–206.

Parsons, T. (1939). The professions and social structure. *Social Forces, 17*(4), 457–467.

Pedersen, A. R. (2008). Narrative identity work in a medical ward: A study of diversity in health care identities. *Tamara: Journal for Critical Organization Inquiry, 7*(1), 38–53.

Reay, T., Goodrick, E., & Hinings, B. (2016). Institutionalization and professionalization. In E. Ferlie et al. (Eds.), *Oxford handbook of health care management* (pp. 25–45). Oxford, UK: Oxford University Press.

Reay, T., Goodrick, E., Waldorff, S. B., & Casebeer, A. (2017). Getting leopards to change their spots: Co-creating a new professional role identity. *Academy of Management Journal, 60*(3), 1043–1070.

Reay, T., & Hinings, C. R. (2009). Managing the rivalry of competing institutional logics. *Organization Studies, 30*(6), 629–652.

Schwartzman, H. B. (1989). *The meeting: Gatherings in organizations and communities.* New York, NY: Plenum Press.

Scott, W. R., Ruef, M., Mendel, P. J., & Caronna, C. A. (2000). *Institutional change and healthcare organizations: From professional dominance to managed care.* Chicago, IL: University of Chicago Press.

Sehested, K. (2002). How new public management challenges the roles of professions. *International Journal of Public Administration, 25*(12), 1513–1537.

Timmermans, S., & Oh, H. (2010). The continued social transformation of the medical profession. *Journal of Health and Social Behavior, 51*(1 supplement), S94–S106.

Weick, K. E. (1979). *The social psychology of organizing.* Reading, MA: Addison-Wesley Publishing.

Wilensky, H. L. (1964). The professionalization of everyone? *American Journal of Sociology, 70*(2), 137–158.

5 Designing and Driving Collaborative, Everyday Innovation Using Narratives

The purpose of this chapter is to investigate how innovative design thinking supports everyday innovation by mobilizing participants and redirecting sensemaking. In most cases of everyday innovation the participants collaborate to solve local problems on their own. In some cases they use design thinking and collaborative design devices from the collaborative innovation literature to support the innovation process. Innovation devices can include collaborative workshops, user pathways, and user narratives. The underlying innovation assumption is that a disruption in everyday routines that introduces, e.g., new external voices, is a design method to innovate and enact change.

The first part of the chapter describes theoretical assumptions in the collaborative innovation literature, especially concerning problem solving via collaborations between external and internal stakeholders. The theme of implementation innovation through the mobilization of participants will also be presented, along with a discussion of the impact of collaborative innovation processes.

The second part of the chapter presents findings from an ethnographic study of two local collaborative innovation projects, both of which concerned empowering patients. The first project was located at a breast cancer ward in a public hospital in the Capital Region, where the innovation project sought to improve the initial medical conversation patients had with health care professionals upon receiving their cancer diagnosis. A local health care innovation center co-designed the plans for the project processes with the ward, bringing in design elements such as patient diaries, focus group interviews, and workshops. This project inspired the development of a new innovation game from the innovation center to be used in all the wards in regional hospitals, creating innovation in the area of improving patient involvement.

The second project was located in a neurology ward at the national hospital in the capital, where the local management group hired a voluntary patient ambassador to design a new project for the ward. The aim of the project was to provide patients with feedback postcards in the waiting areas to write about their perceptions of their patient trajectories while on the ward. The voluntary patient ambassador worked with a group of nurses to design, distribute, and subsequently analyze the postcards. Two additional external participants, a voluntary medical organization for patient safety, and a large private foundation were also part of the change process. This collaboration resulted in the design and conceptualization of a feedback postcard, entirely funded by the foundation and the patient safety organization, for nationwide distribution to provide patient feedback at hospital wards.

The second part of the chapter begins by presenting two shared participant narratives. These narratives supported shared and common understandings of the local values that mobilized participants in the projects. Next, individual participant ante-narratives are presented, which redirected sensemaking of old and new routines about the medical conversation and waiting time, resulting in the creation of new values concerning patient involvement and allowing critical voices to have a legitimate place in the change projects.

The contribution of this chapter is to illustrate how participation in local innovation projects is conditioned upon shared sensemaking and narratives—more concretely, how local values of both external and internal participants are centered around concepts of patient empowerment in everyday innovation processes. The chapter also demonstrates how innovation design devices, such as workshops, focus group interviews, postcards, diaries, and reports can redirect individual sensemaking and illustrate ante-narratives about how to make both critical and positive sense of new waiting room routines and approaches to medical conversations.

Theories of Designing Collaborative Innovation Processes

Theories of designing collaborative innovation processes are derived from various strands of research in governance and collaborative network governance studies (Crosby, 't Hart, & Torfing, 2017; Hartley, Sørensen, & Torfing, 2013; Head & Alford, 2015), public innovation studies (Ferlie, Wood, & Hawkins, 2005; Osborne & Brown, 2011), and innovative design thinking (Bason, 2018; Harris & Albury, 2009).

Many of these innovation studies and traditions build on two classical understandings of innovation. Rogers' (2010) study of innovation described five stages of innovation—knowledge, persuasion, decisions, implementation, and conformation—as linear innovation processes, and Van de Ven, Polley, Garud, and Venkatarman's (1999) innovation studies recognized that innovation processes are not linear but ongoing processes in specific institutional contexts. These two innovation studies represent the episodic and continuous change perspectives (Chapter 3). Many public and organizational studies of innovation build on Andrew Van de Ven et al.'s (1999) understanding of innovation (Ferlie et al.,

2005; Osborne & Brown, 2011; Walker, Berry, & Avellaneda, 2015). In contrast, many innovation design thinking studies build on Rogers's understanding of innovation, defining these phases even more concretely in stages: empathize, define, ideate, prototype, and test (Clarke & Craft, 2019; Harris & Albury, 2009). Collaborative governance studies build on a mixture of these two understandings of innovation by including driver, barrier, and stage understandings of innovation processes and the institutional conditions and context (Crosby et al., 2017; Hartley, 2005; Hartley et al., 2013).

The following chapter will build on Van de Ven et al.'s (1999) understanding of innovation. In *The Innovation Journey*, Van de Ven et al. described the elements that occur during innovation processes: (1) the initiation period, which includes the initiative's innovative ideas; (2) the development period, during which ideas proliferate into numerous activities, including setbacks and parallel understandings of problems; and (3) the implementation period, integrating the new and the old to fit the local situation (p. 24). They illustrated how organizational innovation processes are messy pathways of different activities, where ideas, people, transactions, contexts, and outcomes are seen as important elements rather than in stable, fixed, open-ended, or cumulative stages (p. 8). Context was explained in a macro-view, addressing the macro-structures of technology or industrial infrastructure for innovation (p. 149). In contrast, in the present volume innovation processes are explained from a micro-context view, addressing the local interactions and sensemaking processes of participants in a local everyday organizing context.

Health care innovation is innovation processes in the context of the health care sector. Omachonu and Einspruch (2010) defined health care innovation as, "The introduction of a new concept, idea, service or process, or product aimed at improving, treatment, diagnosis, education, outreach, prevention and research and with the long term of improving quality, safety, outcomes, efficiency and cost" (p. 5). This definition describes the general elements of health care innovation processes that cover both product innovation and service innovation. Hence, the prior definition could also encompass practices beyond the individual organization, including relationships with external organizations and people, in addition to a more network and inter-organizational understanding. Hartley (2005) defined innovation from a governance perspective as a certain kind of innovation, which, also in a health care setting, goes beyond organizational boundaries and creates network-based interactions (Moore & Hartley, 2008). The collaborative innovation literature highlights the importance of including external stakeholders in the innovation processes. The challenge then becomes possibilities of organizing interaction between the participants in these networks, as well as how to create collectively established ideas and goals. Ferlie et al. (2005) concluded in their public innovation studies in a health care context that social interactions, trust, and motivation are important elements in health care change and innovation processes, but they are not always optimal in local contexts (p. 131). Thus collaborative everyday innovation in a health care context can be understood as both product and service innovation and includes collaborations between organizational members and external stakeholders implementing or translating new ideas into everyday routines to create legitimately new impact and values. This means that everyday innovation involves sensemaking negotiations of which problems, goals, and values the innovations should address in a locally situated context, as they cannot be defined beforehand.

Making Sense of Problems and Solutions Via Internal and External Collaboration

Contemporary governance studies emphasize the possibilities of solving complex global issues by addressing complex problems. One claim is that complex problems cannot be solved in hierarchies and through intra-organizational views, as a recent idea in these studies is the important role of the involvement of various external stakeholders in solving complex problems, e.g., by including politicians, citizens, and voluntary organizations (Crosby et al., 2017). The literature argues that public innovation should solve complex global issues, which some researchers consider to be ill-defined and wicked problems (Bommert, 2010; Head & Alford, 2015; Weber & Khademian, 2008). Wicked problems are complex policy problems which must be solved in collaborative networks to provide adequate responses to contemporary challenges, such as climate change, aging societies, or financial crises, which all require broader collaborations. Head and Alford (2015) explored how collaboration assists in dealing with wicked problems by enabling a degree of trust and mutual commitment among the participating parties. This means that to be able to bring diverse types of knowledge together, the participants must have trust in their relationships and find common ground regarding what the problems and the potential solutions are. But practicing collaborative innovation between internal and external participants brings organizational challenges, such as how to involve the many different stakeholders in defining the problem and maintaining a legitimate solution that offers relevant interactions for all stakeholders (Crosby et al., 2017). Just as the collaborative innovation literature notes the importance of including external stakeholders, collaborative everyday innovation happens in everyday routines through the participation of local employees and external stakeholders, with shared problems that make sense to them and can be related to their culturally accepted and legitimate contextual values.

The organizational innovation literature emphasizes the role of narratives, suggesting that values, feelings, and meanings play a key role in creating common ground for social interaction during the innovation process. Narratives have the capability to define identity formation and accepted practices of participation (Coopey, Keegan, & Elmer, 1997; Hjort and Steyaert, 2004; Pedersen, 2016). An innovation study by Hjort and Steyaert (2004) described the importance of sensemaking to the innovation process, and how narratives create shared meaning, directions, and social interactions. Another innovation study by Coopey et al. (1997) studied the role of managers' narratives in sensemaking in an innovation process and concluded that managers are able to creatively draw on their individual memory when composing a story to make sense of what is happening, while potentially enhancing feelings of self-esteem. They also showed how narratives consequently serve to confirm or reshape a manager's identity within the innovation activity (p. 312). In a health care innovation study, Pedersen (2016) illustrated how patient narratives particularly play an important role in creating sense for health care professionals, as patient narratives represent a certain kind of patient experience that supports engagement and participation in the innovation processes. The sensemaking innovation literature highlights the need for participation to include sensemaking processes.

Mobilizing Innovation Participation Via Innovation Designs as User Experiences

In the context of everyday organizing, the processes of generating new ideas are often bound to the quest of solving complex local problems (Pedersen, 2016). As these problems are often very complex to solve and require legitimate approaches in redirecting sensemaking, a new trend has been to introduce design thinking to structure these processes (Bason, 2018). Clarke and Craft (2019) wrote about new trends of using design thinking in the public sector, asserting that new designs are often used with the goal of deliberately improving policy making outcomes, through early, open-ended exploration of problems and solutions and iterative prototyping. Often, design thinking relies on user experience and satisfaction as the primary input into policy design processes. They further offer a critical view of design thinking, arguing that in some cases design thinkers present what they purport to be a superior model of policy-making that is naïve, as it does not include policy design dilemmas and orthodoxy. Clarke and Craft recommended that designers must consider the need for ongoing consistency, coherence, and congruence of policy design, which can be challenged as the design evolves (p. 13). An implication of this view is that design models also evolve in processes and need to make sense for the participants in relation to their everyday routines and their understanding of policy problems.

In a health care context, design thinking often uses the design methods of user experience. As such, patient involvement methods have been a recent design trend in health care (Kjær & Pedersen, 2010; McDermott & Pedersen, 2016), which means that addressing a legitimate policy problem can lead to improved conditions for patients. Pedersen (2016) demonstrated how patient narratives are constructed by including multiple voices of patients and health care professionals. Patient narratives are social constructions (Bury, 2004), which are recorded and retold by researchers, consultants, and health care professionals to become representative accounts (Pedersen, 2016).

One of the problems of translating innovative ideas into everyday routines is the mundane task of mobilizing participants to change routines and persuading them to follow new ideas, when doing so will mean that their work may become more challenging due to new requirements; it does not necessarily remove or reduce old routines. Consequently, innovation can become associated with an increased workload, as new layers of work are added, often leaving participants skeptical or critical of replacing old routines with new ones (Ferlie et al., 2005; Fitzgerald, Ferlie, Wood, & Hawkins, 2002; Veenswijk, 2006).

A study by Mantere and Vaara (2008) investigated conditions of participation in organizational change processes, demonstrating how participation is linked to sensemaking and to broader social discourses. They distinguished between three social discourses that appear to reproduce a non-participatory approach: mystification (the obfuscation of organizational decisions), disciplining (using disciplinary techniques to constrain action), and technologization (imposing a technical system to govern activities) (p. 348). They also identified three social discourses that enhance participation: self-actualization (discourse on the ability to outline objects in the process), dialogization, and concretization (discourse that seeks to establish clear understandings and practices). Consequently, their study demonstrated how certain kinds of social discourses create sensemaking conditions for participation.

In a health care setting, health care professionals are often described as one of the main barriers against change and innovation due to their claim of autonomy and their mono-professional means of organizing hindering collaboration with other professions (Sehested, 2002). This means that the involvement of health care professionals cannot be taken for granted and requires a great deal of work to redirect sensemaking as a condition for participation. The methods of user designs in the health care setting necessitate the inclusion of patient narratives, requiring that new insights are related to existing routines and that the participants negotiate how user experiences add to the political, subjective, normative, and democratic power of defining policy problems (Clark & Craft, 2019).

From an episodic linear innovation perspective, the impact of an innovation's outcome can be measured by whether the degree of activities are of mundane or radical innovation. Innovation is characterized by discontinuity with past routines (Hartley, 2012), with inherently experimental outcomes (p. 173). Hartley argues that many small-scale changes over time can lead to radical shifts in policies and strategies of practice but change processes can also have insufficiently radical or disruptive step-changes to be defined as innovation (p. 177). In contrast, in a continuous innovation approach, the impact of innovation is understood as a change in values or logics, as changing logics, values, and beliefs is a difficult process in innovation and organization (Goodrick & Reay, 2011). This means that the outcome of the innovation processes is related to a redirection of sensemaking (Weick & Quinn, 1999), and one way to do that is by integrating new routines into the old routines.

Partial Discussion and Conclusion

The innovation literature is difficult to present as a coherent collection of ideas, as so many different interpretations and concepts are part of this literature. This chapter attempts to divide the innovation literature into two strands of research: those having a linear understanding of change and innovation, such as design thinking and parts of the governance literature, and those having a processual understanding of innovations, as in organizational and public innovation studies.

When innovation is dominated by a linear design understanding—design advice, ideas for how to solve policy problems, e.g., as collaborations or with designs or representations being given the main attention—it aims to disrupt and advance radical innovation by breaking with old routines.

When innovation is dominated by the understanding of continuous change as everyday innovation it calls for a critical view of design thinking as many design concepts become simplifications and do not stress the complexity of solving policy problems. An everyday innovation context stresses the inclusion of taking situated context into account (Dopson, Fitzgerald, & Ferlie, 2008), wherein design ideas make sense in relation to identified local values. Everyday innovations are not generic but are translated by making sense of local problems in the context of everyday routines. This means that collaborative innovation ideas need to address the organizational setting, as hierarchies do not disappear when seeking collaborative solutions.

Everyday Innovation Through Shared Narratives of Participation and Fragmented Narratives of Representation

The second part of this chapter will demonstrate how both shared and fragmented sensemaking are part of local innovation processes. To begin with, shared or combined narratives of participation capturing collective meanings of groups (Mantere & Vaara, 2008) are presented. The first shared narrative examined concerns engagement and the second one materialization. At the end of the chapter, several ante-narratives are presented that represent participants' individual sensemaking about the old and new routines of waiting and of medical encounters.

The narratives are from two ethnographic studies of collaborative innovation in a breast cancer ward at a regional hospital and a neurology ward at a hospital in the capital region. In the breast cancer ward, a group of local clinical managers (head doctors) decided to invite the regional innovation center to help them to engage the health care professionals in the ward to improve the initial medical conversation. In this conversation, the patient received their cancer diagnosis, and the health care professionals wanted to know the patients' reactions after learning about their diagnosis and how they could improve the conversation to reduce anxiety. To do this they gave the patients diaries to write about their experience. The innovation center introduced design devices from design thinking, including focus group interviews with patients and health care professionals about their diaries and collaborative workshops with the health care professions. In these contexts they made new sense of the patients' experiences and suggested new routines for conducting these conversations.

In the neurology ward, a local clinical manager (a head nurse) decided to invite a patient ambassador, who was a former patient, to talk about the idea of introducing feedback postcards on the ward, which she got after a trip to the US. The local project group, consisting of nurses and the patient ambassador, was established to implement the idea. They had to design the postcard and determine how it should work, where the postcards should be announced and placed, and how they should collect the cards and use them after receiving them. They conducted a pilot project, during which they collected and registered patient feedback to measure the effects of the cards. In the process, members from a private foundation joined the group, as they believed the feedback postcards would also be relevant in other wards.

Both cases are an example of broader collaborations and the use of design elements. Devices from innovation design thinking included: collaborative workshops, focus group interviews, diaries, postcards, pilot projects, and measurement of effects. Each project resulted in culture-changing impact, changing the routines of patients waiting and medical conversations.

The contribution of these findings is to illustrate the emergence of shared sensemaking in health care professionals and certain external participants in situated local health care contexts and to demonstrate how shared sensemaking is a combination of the fragmented sensemaking of patients (as user voices), health care professionals, and other external participants. This leads to a discussion of the relationship between organizational members and external stakeholders in collaborative innovation, the usefulness of design thinking in innovation, and the impact of local innovation projects.

Shared Narratives of Participation

In both of the innovation projects presented earlier, a set of combined or shared narratives from both internal and external participants, which reflected common values, were identified. These common values created motivation to participate in the two projects. The first shared narrative was about patient engagement, as all participants were interested in the joint goal of engaging more with patients to learn from them and patient empowerment was a value they supported. The second shared narrative was about materiality, as the participants stressed that they did not like going to meetings and talking about new projects; instead, they required tangible objects to work with that made the projects concrete. They wanted to work with concrete objects like postcards or diaries.

At the same time, many individual ante-narratives about the innovation projects surfaced. The patient narratives from diaries and postcard did not represent shared or collective meanings, as they brought up many different issues, and the health care professionals' readings and interpretations of the diaries and postcards also resulted in fragmented sensemaking.

Shared Narratives of Engagement in Solving Local Problems

When innovation is initiated in a local ward, defining and understanding the problem and the reasons associated with the innovation project is important, as it is a central theme in making sense of the project. All of the interviewees explained their values concerning patients and why change was necessary, each of them mentioning how increased patient empowerment was important because they worked with the patients daily, but they did not always hear about what the patients experienced during their hospital stay. The interviews described how they discovered that what was important to patients during their stay could stand in contrast to their own ideas and understanding of what patients needed. As one doctor from the diary project stated, "We think we know what they think, but this turns out not to be entirely the case." This statement illustrates the engagement narrative that emerged from the health care professionals, who explained why this project was important and why they should spend their time on it. In the breast cancer ward, the chief physician had participated in a course and had developed an interest in bringing in patient perspectives to improve quality in her ward. Here, she recounted her attempt to make sense of the importance of patient involvement:

> I participated in a qualitative development course and I found that involving the patients was exciting. There was a case about patient involvement from a pharmacy, where the pharmacist involved the customers in the design of the new pharmacy. I found that really interesting. So, I talked a lot about involving the patients more in our work. Then I met with Liz and Monica and we started to talk about it. Monica asked if anyone in the department had any ideas, which was at the same time as the health innovation center started. That was lucky for us. We then searched for a project where we could involve the patients. We thought it was natural to start with the first day they came to the ward and started to ask them about that day. Just because we think we know what patients are like, it doesn't mean it's necessarily like that. We have to ask the patients in order to know.

The chief physician explained how she heard about patient involvement during a course and how she then told everyone in the clinic. The patient ambassador from the postcard project stated:

> I am a spokesperson for patient involvement, which is a battle I take to the doctors. We cannot learn from this without knowing if it is the case 5 or 35 times a year; we try to learn anyway. The patient can point out so many problems that reflect other problems, so, for the individual patient, one communication problem is relevant, but the interesting part is if we ask, "Does this have anything to do with the way we're organized?", that makes us vulnerable to this type of communication.

This example illustrates how engaged support for patient empowerment, which includes listening more to health care system users is central to creating sense of the projects.

Patient empowerment refers to the importance of involving patient knowledge and patient communication as the basis for improving professional treatment and care. In many of the interviews, the health care professionals described how they found patient empowerment interesting, exciting, and motivational, and they agreed on the importance of asking patients about their opinions instead of assuming they knew what they were already. Thus the engagement of patient empowerment was a shared local value that led to an interest in involvement with this project.

Shared Narratives of Materiality in Innovation Designs

In both cases, the interviews talked about the importance of having concrete tools to work with in the innovation process: postcards and diaries. The materiality of the innovation devices helped them to conduct activities around this patient feedback.

In the postcard case, when they were being designed, everyone had an opinion about their design, placement, presentation to patients, and collection and evaluation. The chief nurse made the following comments about the strong effects of working with the postcards:

> I think it's important that the staff on the ward read the postcards, get them in their hands and look at them. It has a much stronger effect when you look at the written word. It's much more personal than looking at statistics. In one ward, the postcards were lying on a desk, freely available where the staff could easily read them. Later, they were put in a folder. I read some postcards where the patients complained about the noise. The head nurse simply had the doors soundproofed without a big discussion or lots of planning. She just did it.

The involved health care professionals explained how the concrete items (postcards) helped them to understand patients' experiences, giving direction to the implementation process. The cards served as something tangible in their sense of the implementation process. The sensemaking about the postcards set the direction of the work tasks involved in the implementation process, e.g., how to design the cards, how to give them to patients, and how to evaluate them when they were filled out and returned. The quote also demonstrates how the patient ante-narratives were not only mental and language devices, but that they also exerted a performative effect: "She just did it." Bartel and Garud (2009) described how narratives have the capacity to coordinate activities in innovation processes, and as in this case, also direct action.

The diaries were supplemented by focus group interviews with patients, during which the content of the diaries was discussed by other patients (after their acceptance). One of the nurses explained why she thoroughly appreciated the focus group interviews as part of the diary project:

> I simply love the focus group interviews. I think I get so must more out of it. I have the possibility to ask more deeply about matters, and I think it's so exiting to do this, to get the possibility to ask about other patient experiences.

She also explained how the combination of diaries and focus groups gave her new reflections and helped her to coherently understand more about what the patients were feeling and thinking after their first medical interviews, when they were given their cancer diagnosis.

Here, the innovation consultant is talking about how the wards worked with the innovation tools in different ways than she sometimes imagined:

> I teach how to use diaries because they want to have diaries. One can ask whether or not that is the right tool for this project. Others will have photo diaries, then I help them with that. . . . In the health service, it's difficult to work with already developed design methods, but there are no tools made more directly for the health care sector.

In this narrative, the innovation consultant expressed how difficult it can be to steer health care professionals, as they are translating the tools into what makes sense for them and therefore not following the "right" innovation design textbooks but understanding designs as practical tools they can use in various activities. Even though the designs did not result in an innovation product (as the consultant would have liked), both cases showed how shared narratives of the materiality—postcards and diaries—were important drivers for engaging health care professionals in the projects.

Summing up, the shared narratives of engagement from the clinical managers and the patient ambassador, and the shared narratives of materiality led to engaged participation in the local innovation projects. They both refer to the social discourses identified in Mantere and Vaara's (2008) participation studies. The first narrative of engagement was related to the social discourse of self-actualization, wherein people like to participate if they can see themselves as part of the project, and they can relate to the object of the project. The second narrative of materialization was related to the social discourse of concretization represented by the diaries and the postcards, as these design elements became tangible objects with clear practices in the projects. Many other narratives of local projects did not create shared sensemaking for the participants; even so, they did result in individual participation.

Redirecting Sensemaking by Individual Ante-Narratives

The innovation processes in both projects resulted in not only shared narratives and sensemaking but also in many individual and more fragmented ante-narratives. One of these included design narratives in the form of patient ante-narratives from the diaries and postcards, described as short and fragmented in both cases (for an ante-narrative framework, see Chapter 2).

Another type of ante-narrative was also presented in the form of the individual narratives of participants that expressed positive and negative feelings about their participation. They were interpretations of the patient ante-narratives and of the change processes, representing many different interpretations of patient ante-narratives as examples of patient experiences. Together, these ante-narratives demonstrate how routines are always sensemaking and negotiated processes in an everyday context, and new interpretations are part of these negotiations when determining how to enact routines.

Design Narratives: Ante-Narratives of Patients in the
Postcards and Diaries

The written patient narratives in the diaries and postcards were surprisingly brief and more fragmented than the health care professionals had imagined they would be. Some were negative, but most were positive. Here are some examples from of the patient ante-narratives on the postcards:

> There's too much commotion in the cramped waiting room and there are not enough chairs.
> I was received kindly and despite the wait, you can always enjoy yourself with a hot drink from the vending machine.

Some of the topics the postcards touched on included the physical environment, communication, and treatment conditions.

> I would like a doctor to contact.
> The professionals work professionally and are always positive. The coffee could be better and the TV in the patient room should be better.
> The professionals have time to listen. A bit of confusion about doing a (treatment) plan and the communication between doctors and nurses could be better to give patients peace of mind.
> The room has not been cleaned!!

The patient ante-narratives were formed by fragmented story work from the diaries and postcards comprising personal accounts of issues they faced while sick along with feelings and encounters with the health care professionals. The writing was surprisingly short, revealing many different feelings and reflections from patients entering the wards. Some postcards praised the professionals by specifically naming good doctors or nurses, but others also criticized people by name. In general, the narratives on the postcards were shorter than expected, mainly listing statements as opposed to describing events at length. (Access to the full patient diaries was not given to the researcher by the innovation center as they collected the patient diaries; instead, fragments of the diaries were available at a workshop.) In general, the health care professionals were caught unaware by the content of the feedback, revealing that patients had many different views that the professionals were unacquainted with. Some of the narratives in the diaries and postcards contained positive and negative elements. The positive narratives shared encouraging statements; the negative ones put forth disapproving statements and had to be handled with more sensitivity by local managers to avoid mistrust and resistance to patient ante-narratives.

Ante-Narratives of Representation

As part of the innovation processes, many activities were involved in the postcards and diaries of the patients: workshops with the health care professionals, focus group interviews with patients and professionals, reports collecting their statements, and a baseline report collecting impact. These activities led to discussions and, in the end, new routines in both wards. The head nurse in the neurological ward read selected postcards at staff meetings, on a daily basis, and decided to solve many of the practical problems raised quickly after reading them. The physicians and nurses at the cancer ward decided to change the topics on the first medical conversation and began offering secondary medical conversations, as they discovered that patient anxiety came several days after diagnosis. Even as these new routines were added, the interpretations of the diaries and postcards as patient representations led to ongoing sensemaking and debates, including both negative and positive ante-narratives.

One of the most critical voices came from the innovation consultant, who was disappointed that the diary project only aimed to improve the first medical conversation. That was not a legitimate innovation goal in the eyes of the innovation consultant, as service design should be more ambitious; she stated: "In my opinion, it's more of a development project than an innovation project. They would just like to improve their communication model. That is, of course, fine, nothing wrong with that, but the innovation goal is not very high."

For the health care professionals at the wards, the medical encounter is one of the most important routines of the ward. Sharing a cancer diagnosis is a medical practice that requires discretion and professional conduct. For the innovation consultant introducing design thinking, this routine is considered to be a communication model, which explains the disappointing relationship between external innovation consultants and health care professionals. The innovation consultant preferred more radical innovations that could be measured more effectively, even though she did not have a full understanding of the local routines and values of the health care professionals.

Some of the most positive ante-narratives came from the health care professionals participating in the workshops and the focus group interviews. One nurse described what an eye-opener reading the post-cards in the workshops were:

> and then there was a relative who described how two nurses, stand-ing across from his wife, criticized some practical physical issues as though his wife was not a human being. That's one you hang on the wall that really makes . . . that gives you pause for thought.

The interviews with health care professionals after the workshops demonstrated how ante-narratives about the diaries and postcards were central to translating the abstract idea of patient empowerment into a concrete, contextual new value of patient empowerment. An experienced chief physician described his reaction to some of the content in the dia-ries, as follows:

> We gave them [patients] diaries. We imagined they were scared. They had just come from tests and other departments and had been diag-nosed with a deadly disease. We gave them an open book. We thought we knew what they were thinking but asked them to write openly about their feelings and their experiences. They did not write much, only a few lines. After the first consultation, they were more relaxed. That surprised us; they had just received some bad news, but they had also received a lot of information that made them feel secure and safe. When interviewed 14 days after their first surgery, that feeling of security was gone and they felt afraid while they were waiting for the results. We gained new information about this waiting time. They did not like it and we have to look at that. I perhaps thought that we could gain more new knowledge about the patients, but we've learned to use these methods so we can ask about more problematic issues next time, for example, the internal communication between the staff.

The health care professionals were surprised by what they read about waiting times in the diary project as well as feelings of insecurity and mistrust. They thought that the first medical conversation would be the worst for patients, but the patients opened professionals' eyes to the fact that it was the second one about their new cancer diagnosis that filled them with the strongest feelings of anxiety.

In the post card case, during its implementation, a private founda-tion felt that the project was so promising that they allocated funding to have the postcards professionally designed and to promote their use nationwide. The health care professionals who participated in the project complained that external requests took attention away from patients and forced them to work with patient data and evaluating the effects of the project. A project nurse spoke about her participation in collecting scien-tific evidence for the project:

> We had to hurry to get the postcards out, so we could measure the effect. That was difficult in the short timeframe we had, but we had to, so [the patient ambassador] could analyze our data to show the effect of the cards.

This quote reflects the unwillingness to measure the impact of the cards, which was perceived as a waste of time and an activity they tried to avoid participating in. Another project nurse described the involvement of the private foundation as follows:

> I was terribly surprised by the direction the project took. I thought it was a qualitative project, but the assessment gives the impression that it was quantitative. How many people said this and how many that? It ended up being more a test involving concepts and design, but I still think the idea is good. . . . I think it shifted ownership.

Despite indications of reluctance from the participants, the focus on scientific quality measurements and external legitimation became an important aspect of validating the project for the foundation, so they participated, even though these activities made little sense to them. The ante-narratives of the participation in reading and understanding of the patient narratives, and the design process illustrated that both positive and negative narratives were emerging. The health care professionals were surprised and changed their perspectives on understanding the patients beforehand; they acknowledged the representation of patient narratives as providing new patient-oriented knowledge. The health care professionals were less impressed by other elements from design thinking. They did not understand the value of testing the results, and the ante-narrative of the innovation consultant demonstrated the different values of design thinking and heath care professions.

The ante-narratives came as a surprise to the health care professionals, as they were so short and fragmented. What they wrote also came as a revelation, as well as how their interpretations of routines differed from the health care professionals' interpretations. In accordance with Hjort and Steyaert (2004), narratives will always generate different types of sensemaking under innovation processes. Some ante-narratives were negative narratives of treatment practices and innovation ambitions, whereas other narratives were positive, generating new insights and facilitating a new understanding of patients. Narrative studies have demonstrated how positive and success narratives often become public and visible, in contrast to negative or failure narratives, which often have a more silent existence, outside of the public eye (Humle & Pedersen, 2014; Vaara, 2002). Here, the negative patient narratives about individuals and the disappointed design narratives were hidden away and became silent narratives.

Discussion and Conclusion

These findings demonstrate how collaborative innovative processes include both internal partners and external stakeholders. In the postcard case the patient ambassador became one of the most important participants, working in trustful relations with the health care professionals, as they shared common local values of patient empowerment. In the diary case the innovation consultant never fully understood the values of the health care professionals and became disappointed over the project, as the results did not match the values of the design thinking literature. Consequently, collaborations between internal health care professionals and external stakeholders are related to shared narratives of participation.

The findings further illustrate how health care professionals are motivated by internal feelings and values. Involvement can be related to a particular internal professional identity and feelings of self-esteem (Coopey et al., 1997), wherein patient empowerment becomes a contextual shared value that creates self-esteem. The ethnographic approach made it possible to investigate the local values of patient empowerment by hearing the narratives and analyzing both the shared and more fragmented individual ante-narratives.

The first narrative analysis demonstrated how shared narratives of engagement and materialization are important elements in mobilizing participants in local innovation projects and how they related to the social discourses of self-actualization and concretization (Mantere & Vaara, 2008, p. 347). According to Mantere and Vaara (2008), discipline can be a non-participatory approach, but in the postcard case perhaps the nurses participated in collecting data because of a strong sense of discipline concerning scientific legitimation, even though they expressed frustration and a loss of meaning concerning this type of participation. This analysis demonstrates how local, contextual, cultural values, such as patient empowerment, become sensemaking drivers of innovation. Furthermore, this analysis demonstrates how innovative designs, such as postcards, diaries, and workshops, create materiality and allow for individual sensemaking, not in the form that was intended (in the design literature) but in ways that create sense for the participants. Acknowledging narratives as sensemaking devices, this analysis demonstrates how both shared and fragmented narratives are linked to a willingness to be involved and to resist (Laine & Vaara, 2007; Levy, Alvesson, & Willmott, 2003). The second narrative analysis demonstrated that the patient ante-narratives were a surprise, as they identified alternative interpretations and were short and fragmented. The health care professionals were taken aback by the content of the feedback, which revealed that patients had many different views that the professionals were unacquainted with. The patient narratives and design tools demonstrated both negative and positive narratives. While the health care professionals were surprised by the patient ante-narratives, they were positive when reading them and willing to include them and use them to redirect their sensemaking of patients. They were more negative toward other design tools, and the innovation consultant was disappointed in the way they used the tools. Negative ante-narratives also emerged about the value of design thinking.

Finally, these analyses show how everyday innovation processes can be "disappointing design innovation projects" in the eyes of an innovation consultant, as their impact was related to a redirecting of values and sensemaking, taking into account the everyday organizing contexts. These elements are difficult to measure from the perspective of design thinking devices, and therefore collaborative innovation also calls for a "collaboration" between organizational and public innovation theories and design thinking theories, setting local innovation projects free from mainstream design values and conventional linear innovation thinking.

References

Bartel, C. A., & Garud, R. (2009). The role of narratives in sustaining organizational innovation. *Organization Science, 20*(1), 107–117.

Bason, C. (2018). *Leading public sector innovation: Co-creating for a better society*. Oxford, UK: Policy Press.

Bommert, B. (2010). Collaborative innovation in the public sector. *International Public Management Review, 11*(1), 15–33.

Bury, M. (2004). Researching patient-professional interactions. *Journal of Health Services Research & Policy, 9*(1 supplement), 48–54.

Clarke, A., & Craft, J. (2019). The twin faces of public sector design. *Governance, 32*(1), 5–21.

Coopey, J., Keegan, O., & Elmer, N. (1997). Managers' innovations as "sensemaking". *British Journal of Management, 8*(4), 301–315.

Crosby, B. C., 't Hart, P., & Torfing, J. (2017). Public value creation through collaborative innovation. *Public Management Review, 19*(5), 655–669.

Dopson, S., Fitzgerald, L., & Ferlie, E. (2008). Understanding change and innovation in healthcare settings: Reconceptualizing the active role of context. *Journal of Change Management, 8*(3–4), 213–231.

Ferlie, E., Fitzgerald, L., Wood, M., & Hawkins, C. (2005). The (non) spread of innovations: The mediating role of professionals. *The Academy of Management Journal, 48*(1), 117–134.

Fitzgerald, L., Ferlie, E., Wood, M., & Hawkins, C. (2002). Interlocking interactions, the diffusion of innovations in health care. *Human Relations, 55*(12), 1429–1449.

Goodrick, E., & Reay, T. (2011). Constellations of institutional logics: Changes in the professional work of pharmacists. *Work and Occupations, 38*(3), 372–416.

Harris, M., & Albury, D. (2009). The innovation imperative. *NESTA*. Retrieved from https://media.nesta.org.uk/documents/the_innovation_imperative.pdf

Hartley, J. (2005). Innovation in governance and public services: Past and present. *Public Money and Management, 25*(1), 27–34.

Hartley, J. (2012). Public value through innovation and improvement. In J. Benington & M. H. Moore (Eds.), *Public value: Theory and practice* (pp. 171–184). Basingstoke, UK: Palgrave Macmillan.

Hartley, J., Sørensen, E., & Torfing, J. (2013). Collaborative innovation: Available alternative to market competition and organizational entrepreneurship. *Public Administration Review*, *73*(6), 821–830.

Head, B. W., & Alford, J. (2015). Wicked problems: Implications for public policy and management. *Administration & Society*, *47*(6), 711–739.

Hjort, D., & Steyaert, C. (2004). *Narrative and discursive approaches in entrepreneurship*. Cheltenham, UK: Edward Elgar.

Humle, D. M., & Pedersen, A. R. (2014). Fragmented work stories: Developing an antenarrative approach by discontinuity, tensions and editing. *Management Learning*, *4*(5), 582–597.

Kjær, P., & Pedersen, A. R. (Eds.). (2010). *Ledelse gennem patienten: Nye styringsformer i sundhedsvæsenet*. Copenhagen, DK: Handelshøjskolens Forlag.

Laine, P. M., & Vaara, E. (2007). Struggling over subjectivity: A discursive analysis of strategic development in an engineering group. *Human Relations*, *60*(1), 29–58.

Levy, D. L., Alvesson, M., & Willmott, H. (2003). Critical approaches to strategic management. In M. Alvesson & H. Willmott (Eds.), *Studying Management Critically* (2nd ed., pp. 92–110). London: Sage.

Mantere, S., & Vaara, E. (2008). On the problem of participation in strategy: A critical discursive perspective. *Organization Science*, *19*(2), 341–358.

McDermott, A. M., & Pedersen, A. R. (2016). Conceptions of patients and their roles in healthcare: Insights from everyday practice and service improvement. *Journal of Health Organization and Management*, *30*(2), 194–206.

Moore, M., & Hartley, J. (2008). Innovations in governance. *Public Management Review*, *10*(1), 3–20.

Omachonu, V. K., & Einspruch, N. G. (2010). Innovation in healthcare delivery systems: A conceptual framework. *The Innovation Journal: The Public Sector Innovation Journal*, *15*(1), 1–20.

Osborne, S. P., & Brown, L. (2011). Innovation, public policy and public services delivery in the UK: The word that would be king? *Public Administration*, *89*(4), 1335–2011.

Pedersen, A. R. (2016). The role of patient narratives in healthcare innovation: Supporting translation and meaning making. *Journal of Health Organization and Management*, *30*(2), 244–257.

Rogers, E. M. (2010). *Diffusion of innovations* (4th ed.). New York: The Free Press.

Sehested, K. (2002). How new public management challenges the roles of professionals. *International Journal of Public Administration*, *25*(12), 1513–1537.

Vaara, E. (2002). On the discursive construction of success/failure in narratives of post-merger integration. *Organization Studies*, *23*(2), 211–248.

Van de Ven, A. H., Polley, E., Garud, R., & Venkatarman, S. (1999). *The innovation journey*. Oxford, UK: Oxford University Press.

Veenswijk, M. (2006). New public management, innovation, and the non-profit domain: New forms of organizing and professional identity. In M. Veenswijk (Ed.), *Organizing innovation: New approaches to cultural change and intervention in public sector organizations* (pp. 10, 15). Oxford, UK: IOS Press.

Walker, R. M., Berry, F. S., & Avellaneda, C. N. (2015). Limits on innovativeness in local government: Examining capacity, complexity, and dynamism in organizational task environments. *Public Administration*, *93*(3), 663–683.

Weber, E. P., & Khademian, A. M. (2008). Wicked problems, knowledge challenges, and collaborative capacity builders in network settings. *Public Administration Review*, *68*(2), 334–349.

Weick, K. E., & Quinn, R. E. (1999). Organizational change and development. *Annual Review of Psychology*, *50*(1), 361–386.

6 Organizational Change Through Narratives of Administrative Coordination

The purpose with this chapter is to illuminate the reconceptualization of the theoretical understanding of coordination that has taken place and show how shared narratives of politicians and administrators become a sensemaking condition for coordination between health care providers. The findings in this chapter are not an example of an everyday innovation initiated from the ward level. Instead, it is an example of how organizational change in health care is also being initiated from the top down as legislation. Thus, a main argument is that sensemaking conditions are relevant for both bottom up as well as top-down change processes through new demands for coordination, as shown in this concrete case. So we are leaving the hospital ward level and moving on to other health care organizations: in this case, the administrative and political steering context. Politicians and administrative employees in the regional offices have the task of coordinating health care services across health care providers and through institutional consolidation. They were merging specialized treatment facilities and making agreements on the tasks assigned to the individual health care providers. Obtaining a license to operate within a public health care system probably carries similar prestige to obtaining a license to kill. Whether the health care system is public or private, politicians and administrators are involved in different ways in prioritizing and coordinating health care services between providers.

Coordination is probably the most cited word when politicians talk about health care systems. Many politicians dream of a health care system in which patients flow naturally from one service provider to another. The dream is a health care system in which coordination is not a challenge, does not present the problem of patients meeting many different health care providers on their individual pathways, and professional autonomy and knowledge specialization does not result in divisions that make collaboration difficult. They desire a system in which specialization and coordination walk hand in hand. This coordination dream indicates a theoretical understanding of coordination balanced with universal force that exists in a golden future. The present, in which coordination is a struggle, is often a complicated effort, a goal for many recent health care policies and reforms to achieve through fixes.

The first section of this chapter presents three different organizational theories of coordination, from a classical design model toward an understanding of contemporary coordination by presenting the concept of pluricentric coordination, wherein many health care providers see themselves as the center of coordination.

In the second part of the chapter an ethnographic study of a health care policy reform will be presented. The goal of the policy reform was to introduce health agreements as a better way to coordinate patient trajectories between health care organizations in regions and municipalities. The regions are the responsible agents for hospitals and general practices, and the municipalities are responsible agents for elderly care, social care, and rehabilitation. The idea with the new policy of health agreements was to enhance coordination and coherence in health care services among local and regional health care service providers. The concept of health agreements was introduced in the health care act of 2007 and had a duration of two years before a new contract was made. Health agreements replaced the previous health plans that each region was using before 2007, describing the region's population in regard to health-related problems and challenges. The first generation of health agreements described certain areas with known coordination problems: hospital discharge processes for weak and elderly patients, rehabilitation plans, assistive aids, and efforts concerning mental disorders. Each region could adjust the effort to local problems, and the agreements were to be crafted by the local health coordination committee (SKU), which included local regional politicians, politicians from municipalities, and representatives from the union of general practitioners as members. Finally, all agreements had to be approved by the National Board of Health. The study followed the work of making the health agreements in the different types of committees, with regional politicians and administrators working together with health care representatives from municipalities, local GPs, and health care representatives from hospitals.

The chapter sets out to illustrate how new demands for coordination as a managerial example of organizational change are conditioned on sensemaking and narratives. The use of everyday ethnography permits an understanding of the routines of local authorities because administrators, politicians, and health care providers meet to negotiate new understandings of coordination.

Theories of Coordination

Traditional organizational studies of coordination were based on the presumption that coordination is the outcome of processes within coherent institutionally or functionally demarcated units that follow a specific, predetermined, and rational logic of consequentiality. In recent years, this unitary, rationalist understanding of coordination has been challenged by a more pluricentric understanding of coordination. Here, coordination is viewed as a messy and floating process that revolves around situated arenas that promote sensemaking between a plurality of values and situated practices. While the traditional theories of coordination tended to view vertical and horizontal forms of coordination as radically different modes of coordination, the new theories question the analytical value of this distinction, emphasizing the relational and interpretive aspects of coordination processes, including the processes by which public health authorities seek to govern their subjects (Pedersen, Sehested, & Sørensen, 2011). The next three sections will present how functional, institutional, and discursive and relational understandings of coordination have developed in organizational studies[1] and represent a main historical development of our understanding of coordination throughout time.

Functional Studies of Coordination

When depicting a hospital as a pyramid diagram, with vertical and horizontal connections to units, we are using a functional description. The focus is on the single organization and our attention is drawn to the structural design of how top management can coordinate with lower levels and how the units of the organization can work together through new regulations and plans. In early studies of organizations, the focus was on single institutions, which could be optimized through studies of workplace conditions, management rules, and personnel conditions. Scientific studies of management were partly pursued by managers and partly by researchers investigating the machinery of organizations (Taylor, 1949). They experimented with the coordination of work through different patterns of work division, standardization, and direct supervision. These studies lay the groundwork for organizational design studies (Pedersen et al., 2011). These design studies, which exclusively focused on intra-organizational coordination, viewed planning as the best way to provide coherent and effective coordination (Fayol, 1949). In this theoretical context, planning was defined as the programmed and strictly regulated distribution of tasks following specific rules (Perrow, 1967). Van de Ven and Delbecq (1976) explained how coordination through planning was established through preexisting plans, schedules, formalized rules, policies, procedures, and standardized information that served as a blueprint for action (p. 323). Thompson (1967) described how these kinds of strictly regulated and programmed actions were formally prescribed in impersonal standards and how these standards needed a minimum of verbal communication because they are implemented as mechanisms of coordination that are codified between task and performers. The design studies paid much attention to the presence of vertical as well as horizontal patterns of coordination, as both were viewed as crucial for ensuring a high level of communization within an organization. The role of ensuring vertical communication was placed on the shoulders of line managers and unit supervisors in general (Pedersen et al., 2011; Thompson, 1967).

The traditional design approach to organizational coordination was redefined with the emergence of Lindblom's (1959) new model on how to understand decisions. Before this, decisions were seen as rational choices. Lindblom's work is based on an understanding that decisions are made by muddling through. Lindblom pointed out the irrational aspects of decisions and coordination. This approach became the basis for future institutional theory. But the period prior to the emergence of contingency theory was a new period, with influence on the understanding of coordination represented by the works of Mintzberg (1983, 1992). His contributions to organizational literature set a new stage for organization theory. He refined the design debate by noting that different kinds of tasks called for different types of organizational forms, each characterized by particular coordination mechanisms in which particular patterns of standardization played a central role (Pedersen et al., 2011). Mintzberg (1983) identified five distinct, ideal typical organizational forms (the entrepreneurial, the machine, the professional, the divisional, and the innovative organization). The concept of the professional organizations, rely on standardization of knowledge, and another, the machine organization, relies on standardization of work. Mintzberg argued that all the types of organizations can be coordinated by means of the following coordination mechanisms: mutual adjustment, direct supervision, and standardization of work, outputs, skills, and norms (Mintzberg & Westley, 1992). While the first one can be characterized as a horizontal form of coordination, the others can be seen as vertical. He argued that only small organizations can rely on horizontal coordination, while large organizations must rely heavily on vertical forms of coordination (Pedersen et al., 2011). A blueprint of a hospital's culture is not a static image, but rather it produces beliefs of order, hierarchy, and control. It also gives the viewer some idea of the coordination issues, including horizontal coordination between subunits, drawing attention to horizontal coordination problems.

Institutional Studies of Coordination

Around the late 1980s, emergence of neo-institutionalism challenged the design tradition in organization theory (March & Olsen, 1989; Meyer & Rowan, 1977; Scott, 1987). Contributors were against the idea that organizations can be studied as isolated islands, placing emphasis on the study of organizational fields and inter-organizational relations as core elements in understanding coordination. They directed the focus of attention toward the role of meaning in coordinating collective action, within as well as between organizations. In other words, the institutionalists moved the focus of attention from coordination through planning, top-down leadership, and standards to how particular institutionalized logics of appropriateness guided behavior, recognizing that the coordination capacity of these informal logics of appropriateness and norms provided the most effective coordination mechanism of all. As these logics are endogenously produced in and through the coordination process itself, each organization developing its particular institutionalized rationalities that serve as mental coordination universes (Pedersen et al., 2011). Consequently, it is a waste of time to seek to develop one universal ideal type of coordination structure. Coordination is produced in different ways in different situations that are driven by particular logics and meanings (Friedland & Alford, 1991; Thornton, Ocasio, & Lounsbury, 2012). Curiously enough, the neo-institutionalist wave resulted in an abundance of both micro- and macro-level analyses, investigating the dominant institutional logics of contemporary organizations (Borum, 2004; Waldorff, Reay, & Goodrick, 2013). One of the effects of these studies was an increased recognition of the loosely coupled nature of organizations—a term which was developed by Orton and Weick (1990). They defined loose couplings in dialectical terms as an act of balancing the oppositional forces of connectivity and autonomy, arguing that too much concern had been directed toward the dangers of structural disconnectedness, thereby overlooking the fact that loose couplings can in fact be of crucial value in the pursuit of coordination within and between organizations (Pedersen et al., 2011). This image of hospitals draws our attention to coordination problems between institutional fields, visualizing similar hospitals with a tendency to look alike, which can be tightly coupled or more loosely coupled.

Discursive and Relational Studies of Coordination

Many new paths have come from the ideas and concepts of neo-institutionalism. One such path has led to theories of sensemaking that direct full attention toward the production of meaning that helps to structure the relationship between the involved actors and gives direction to future actions (Weick, 1993, p. 635). Weick suggested that respectful interaction depends on the presence of intersubjectivity, which: (1) provides an exchange and synthesis of meaning between two or more communicative selves, and (2) transforms the self in the interactive process in a way that adds to the development of shared subjectivity (p. 642). The focus on the development of joint sensemaking placed ongoing interaction and communication at the heart of the coordination process. As such, this line of theorizing has produced a view on coordination being provided upside down—away from standardized and instrumentalized, top-down coordination and more closely to loosely coupled moments of situated sensemaking (Pedersen et al., 2011). In the late 1990s, scholars began to examine the issue of how communication processes accommodated coordination (Boden, 1994; Fairhurst & Putnam, 2004; Quinn & Dutton, 2005). A certain position in this line of research was taken by narrative theory, which views narratives as a particularly forceful form of organizing that illustrates interaction and meaning emerging through narratives (Czarniawska & Joerges, 1997; Gabriel, 2000; Pedersen et al., 2011). From this point of view, narratives within organizations do not, per se, produce a shared, coherent, and consistent universe of meanings.

Rather it is a complex plurality of loosely coupled narratives wherein both individual and shared ante-narratives make sense of the daily experiences in organizations through processes that are not far from the informal horizontal exchanges of information, which Mintzberg (1983) called mutual adjustments, taking place in everyday organizing.

Toward a New Understanding of Coordination

A recent coordination approach is based on the assumption that coordination efforts take place in unstable, undecidable terrain riddled with battles for power and fragmentation (Pedersen et al., 2011; Sørensen, Sehested, & Pedersen, 2011). In this context, the ambition of coordination is defined modestly as an effort to establish relatively fixed moments that make it possible to act collectively. Hence, our understanding of coordination brings into view the already well-established assumption that the continuous capacity to adapt to changing circumstances is crucial to the ability to coordinate. The need to drop the image of coordination as the act of stabilizing or controlling action through the identification of a model of coordination is not only caused by its proven lack of effectiveness. It is also caused by a theoretical recognition of the valuable contributions of flexibility, autonomy, diversity, and complexity for coordination (Pedersen et al., 2011).

The new coordination approach represents a novel layer in the understanding of coordination, placed on top of the three previous conceptions, which develop from a focus on control and coherence to a focus on loose couplings and sensemaking in complex unstable organizing, as represented in Table 6.1:

Table 6.1 Theoretical Approaches to Coordination

	Functional, design	Institutional	Discursive, relational
RATIONALITY	Logic of consequences	Logic of appropriateness	Several logics, interpretative
MECHANISM	Vertical or horizontal	Loose couplings	Interactions
ORGANIZATION	Standards	Norms and values	Sensemaking and narratives

The first stage is represented by functional theories of coordination that proposed a universal approach to coordination. These theories shared the view that coordination is an outcome of a regulation of the actions of actors and processes that are driven by a universal logic of consequentiality. This regulation is carried out through a combination of vertical and horizontal forms of regulation. At the second stage of theory development, criticism was raised against the idea that it is possible to develop a universal model of coordination, with emphasis placed on the need to consider contextual factors, such as institutionalized norms, rules, and practices, which were believed to have a profound impact on coordination processes. The theories began to focus on the loosely coupled relationship between different parts of an organization, and the many internal de-couplings and external factors that disintegrate the organization and undermine its boundaries. At the third stage of theory development, coordination is increasingly perceived as consisting of a patchwork of overlapping meanings that are interacting in non-centralized processes in which different participants seek meanings (Pedersen et al., 2011).

So what are the main ingredients in a narrative approach toward recently developed theories of coordination? Coordination can be defined as situated interactions that promote shared sensemaking between otherwise disconnected narratives. Coordination is situated because it always takes place within a context of change. This is particularly relevant today, as change is now regarded as an unavoidable organizing condition. Interactions are ongoing adjustments with the aim of establishing shared sensemaking of coordination between disconnected narratives. This implies that shared narratives also play an important part in coordination and coordination can be established by many (polyphonic) shared narratives of coordination. What does this development mean for our understanding of coordination? First, coordination understandings and narratives have to be investigated in certain organizing contexts. Second, interaction to reach shared understandings depends on trustful relations, wherein the participants share some kind of local values. Last, coordination through shared narratives represents time sensitive and sensemaking constellations, which can be turned into discoordination or lack of responsibility to engage.

Partial Discussion and Conclusion

This theoretical section provided an overview on organizational coordination and how coordination has been described through functional, institutional, and discursive approaches. The various views have different core concepts: horizon and vertical coordination, loosely coupled institutional fields, and shared understandings and narratives. All of these theories of coordination remain relevant and present in contemporary empirical studies of coordination. A narrative approach toward coordination underlines the importance of shared sensemaking and narratives and how this can be reached when trustful interactions based on shared local values become part of the negotiations and routines of coordination. Mutual adjustment is a concept from Mintzberg (1983) that is still relevant to a narrative approach, in which rules and regulations are not enough for effective coordination.

Shared Narratives of Politicians and Administrators: Making Mutual Adjustments in Health Agreements

The purpose of the second part of this chapter is to demonstrate how shared narratives become a way to make agreements on how to coordinate between regional health care providers.

The findings are from an organizational ethnography of the work that one region and 17 municipalities engaged in when implementing the first generation of health agreements. With 17 municipalities attached to one region, the health agreements were a new policy steering instrument. The study consisted of observations of the SKUs and the ad hoc working groups, as well as interviews with the members of the committees and the regional administers who visited the 17 municipalities to set up the new collaboration for making health agreements.

Before the introduction of the law on health care agreements, the relations between the health care providers in regions (specialized care) and municipalities (rehabilitation and social care) could be characterized as having an atmosphere that was colored with mistrust and stereotypical stories of the unprofessional culture of the counterparts (Mikkelsen, Petersen, & Pedersen, 2016). Narratives of how hospitals were discharging elderly patients on Friday afternoons, after the municipality's care facilities were closed, forcing elderly patients to go home without any assistance, were dominant narratives among the municipalities. Narratives of how the local rehabilitation of patients was of low quality were the dominant narratives from the hospitals (Mikkelsen et al., 2016). The municipal and regional health care professionals also had a shared distrust of the politicians and administrators in the regions, as they were referring to state and corporate logic in contrast to professional health care logic (see Chapter 3). The regional and municipal politicians also mistrusted each other, as they were competing over health care services. In this organizational context we collected narratives from the different committee members as they had to revise and address their storytelling about their former "enemies." We sought to uncover the emergence of new shared narratives that addressed the local solutions of the coordination problems mentioned in the national health agreements policy paper (Sørensen et al., 2011).

The findings are presented through three shared narratives of the politicians and administrators regarding their work on implementing health agreements. The first one described secured operations as a shared value guiding their work in coordination. The next one was the shared value of equal partnership as a new narrative of the relationship between municipalities and regions. Finally, a shared narrative of control is presented, demonstrating that not all the storytelling is based on happy and epic narratives but also on how more critical narratives arise. Together these narratives became some of the dominant narratives of the coordination work in the committees, when, for the first time, they had to establish shared meanings regarding the problems of coordination in health care. One example of coordination problems they discussed was the discharge of patients who subsequently also needed immediate municipal care and making sure that these patients did not fall through the cracks in their transition from hospital care to municipal care.

The contribution of these sections is to demonstrate the kinds of shared narratives that emerged in the new work relationships between regions and municipalities, in which they have to solve concrete coordination problems to implement health agreements, and to demonstrate how shared sensemaking becomes a condition for effective coordination. The first shared narratives resulted in concrete coordination activities.

A Shared Narrative of Secured Operations

The mayors and politicians in the regions and the municipalities have different budgets and different formal tasks in relation to health care services. Coordination of health care is not a hot local political topic, like schools or elderly homes, so the first task was to define the health agreements as either political contracts or administrative service delivery contracts. The politicians from the municipalities had their own shared meeting forum with all of the mayors from the surrounding regional municipalities to select the members for the heath coordination committee. The mayors were not used to representing other mayors or municipalities, so this quickly redirected the work to be about making a new administrative implementation service delivery contract that required new local policy strategies or campaigns. This means that the SKU made up of political members became a formal committee, while all of the work of implementing the health agreements was pushed to lower level committees.

One of the first challenges that came about was figuring out the level of political or strategic goals that the regional and the municipal representatives brought with them. As the coordination of the SKU and the lower level committees was administered by the region initially, the need to focus on secured operations as a legitimate administrative concern that both the municipality and the region could agree on was introduced. The director of the region said:

> When I hear from my colleagues in other regions, I believe this region is the region that runs most painlessly. This means that running operations painlessly matters and brings an important value. This creates a pragmatic view on the health agreements and how they can run and become a success by working painlessly.

Running painlessly can also be translated as avoiding conflicts and thereby the first premise for the new collaboration between regions and municipalities was to avoid conflicts and "pain" to secure the daily operations. The leader of the regional administrative steering committee also added to this:

> You can say it like this. We did this successfully by working forward and by constantly having the possibility of taking action. Our goal is to secure the daily operations and we refuse to introduce goals that will make the task more difficult. Retrospectively, I believe that these two things meant that we could maintain it at a practical, successful level.

Securing the daily operations made it possible to avoid big battles about new political strategies, which is why the SKU used a National Board of Health policy paper to direct the work, instead of translating the general policy problems into a locally driven policy process to address the most local health issues. Using this policy paper also supported the administrative process instead of making it politically driven. As one of the administrative workers from the National Board of Health explained:

> One can say, in the white paper, the topic is just a guiding proposal, and we argue for the background on why these areas were chosen, and we were trying to frame these problems in the paper. But with the response we got back, they told us from the regions that we indicated the right area where many of the problems can be found.

The administration chose a tight coupling with the National Board of Health to make sure that it approved their contract by working with coordination issues they had chosen, instead of working with locally selected problems.

In the ad hoc working group of health care professionals, they accepted this vision for their work, making detailed delivery plans, but they also had broad ambitions and wanted to change some of the existing routines by devising new service delivery routines. But this group was met with the advice that they had to make concrete, detailed plans for delivery before they began building new castles in the sky. The secure operation narrative led to work tasks, wherein detailed plans for delivery were defined as the successful output. The need for successful collaboration between municipalities and regions was deemed more important than implementing new practices for the patients.

Coordination was based on shared sensemaking and narratives about making health agreements to secure operations. This involved asking ad hoc groups (of health care professionals) to make detailed delivery plans for work division and the standardization of work tasks. The health care professionals accepted their role, even though they also asked for a more progressive coordination strategy, but the need to achieve a successful coordination narrative was deemed of primary importance. As such, coordination was guided by a shared narrative of secure operations, which led to the formal organization of vertical and horizontal work delivery plans that did not take into account preexisting problems of why these coordination lines did not always work in practice.

A Shared Narrative About Equal Partnership

Another narrative closely related to the first emerged. This shared narrative addressed the new attempt to work together and tried to reduce the poor relationship between the regions and the municipalities from the past. As regions have responsibility for GPs and hospitals they normally acted as the most important local health care service provider. But, as the municipalities had taken over the responsibility for rehabilitation and local health care delivery to prevent, instead of treat, illnesses, the municipalities acted as if they were now the most important health care service provider.

All of the interviews with politicians and administrators concerned this relationship between municipalities and regions happening through an equal partnership. The head secretary of the region talked about how this notion had to be worked from the beginning:

> We used our network a lot. How should we address that the SKU [health coordination committee], from the beginning, was made up of three members from the region and five from the municipalities, but then we received information from the other regions that they had set up a standing committee with five members from each side. This is a higher degree of coordination than we are used to.

The problem of one region working and collaborating with many municipalities (in this case 17) involved how to divide power in the SKUs between the two public sectors. They found a local solution to prevent the municipality, due to their size, from overruling the region. This example demonstrated how the collaboration was a difficult task, and the region director stated:

> The aim was to get barriers to go down, and to let the new conversations lead to new understandings, where we learn about each other's conditions and problems and that makes it easier when we talk about concrete matters, also about tough issues, when we have to make deals, when money is involved.

He also stated that the regions were no longer the boss in relation to the municipalities, commenting:

Our viewpoint is that we have an equal collaboration.

This new approach stressed that the two service providers should col-laborate instead of competing. A representative from the association of the municipalities talked about the municipality's viewpoint, saying:

Now we're practicing and we can see what kind of partner we're talking with. It won't be a big brother, little sister relationship, but equal partners.

The SKU became a new link between regions and municipalities, and a forum for trustful coordination. A regional Danish People's Party politi-cian, chair of the social committee, and member of the SKU, talked about her first SKU meeting:

It is important that if the municipalities are unhappy with something, or if the regions are unhappy with something, that we have enough confidence to tell each one another and say things directly. We had rehabilitation problems before, but now this has been solved. So, we know what we have to do.

She described how the committee became a new meeting place where they could discuss and solve problems. They all stressed the importance of building up an equal partnership. The only challenge mentioned was when the conversation went from good intentions to hardcore financial negotiations, which was rarely a pretty picture.

These shared narratives of politicians and administrators illustrated how coordination becomes pluricentric, as they abandon the idea of one center of authority for several centers of authority. Both the region and the municipalities are legitimate centers of coordination, which left the SKU to become a meeting place to discuss and make shared sense of the needs and problems due to the lack of coordination between the health service providers. Trust became a central part of these new dialogues. The division of work, however, remained a part of their understanding of coordination, as the last quote states, as previously, that the region and the municipalities had problems with dividing responsibility for rehabili-tation, with the 2007 law specialized rehabilitation is the responsibility of regions, while less specialized rehabilitation is the responsibility of municipalities. The politicians mentioned in relation to that change, that now they know what to do to jointly to solve coordination issues.

A Shared Narrative of Control

In contrast to the narratives of patient and health care professionals, the politicians, and particularly the administrators put forth similar narratives about the legitimate need for a secure operation as an administrative task, which they extended to the political agenda. The politicians also talked about creating trust in environments characterized by political struggle. But not all narratives were positive, happy frontstage narratives. More critical narratives emerged about how to balance between political issues, which should not interfere with securing operations, but should still be concrete and relevant for voters to recognize. The way both politicians and administrators handled this concern was through a shared narrative of control, i.e., shared critical narratives of a top-down culture in both the political environments and in the administrative culture.

Because making health agreements was a new work task for both the politicians and the administrators, they struggled with how to be part of the change process. The politicians' new roles were not to go into the minutia of running the operations, or more concretely, the administrators were trying to keep the politicians away from the daily operations, even though normal political practice was to be involved in individual cases. As an administrative head shared:

> Trying to get a focus on the political and strategic issues and less on the daily operations has been interesting. So, you have the chance to embark on boarder political debates.

He also further described the relationship between himself and the regional chair (a politician):

> I think it's developed. In the beginning, I misunderstood my role, taking what he said as the law. But he asked me to ask questions and he wanted more of a dialogue, and that has developed over time.

A regional politician from a liberal political party stated:

> We have a very strong mayor, and the mayor's management style made me feel like I was back in the National Guard.

By comparing the political management style to that of a military body, she indicates that it was very formal and top-down oriented. She also described work in the SKU, during which, as part of the meeting agenda, they discussed strategies involving the coordination of discharging patients from the hospitals. She preferred a more political agenda that was related more to her voters. She said:

> Yes, but the key [in the discharge process] involves the chief physician because the chief physician on the ward is the one who tells Miss Hansen that she is ready [and needs to go home] . . . and the hospitals cannot survive with bad stories in the press. . . . But, we

want to have a piece of the cake too, to make us visible and to have agenda such as wellness, which is a new business opportunity in the region that we can go out and tell the press about to make ourselves more visible on television.

In this account, she placed all responsibility for coordinating the discharge process into the hands of the hospital, leaving room for a loose coupling, even though the municipalities would also like to have avoided the application of some discharge rules, e.g., not on Friday afternoons, for certain kinds of patients. She further addressed that she would like to discuss broader themes that are more press-oriented, such as wellness, which, in comparison with discharge coordination, is a more attractive political agenda.

The head of regional financing talked about their internal discussion on agenda setting at SKU meetings:

I feel like there's a lot of control over the process, where the chair is in control and knows what's going on. I wasn't used to very much control before. They even corrected commas in my internal agenda notes.

Together, these statements paint a picture of a regional culture in which political groups struggled over agendas, so the role of formal political leadership dictated the agenda setting in a controlling way. Both politicians and administrators talked about top-down steering, where the shared narratives of secure operations and an equal partnership controlled the meeting agendas. The previous quotes also demonstrate the difficulties involved in the politicians being concerned with regional coordination at the hospital level, as the regional political culture was described in terms of a battle about suitable political agendas and emphases. These combined narratives portray a controlling and formal political culture, where coordination follows the shared narratives of secure operation but via controlled agenda setting. These more critical narratives raise the problematic issues concerning trust in relation to control and how control can become the solution in a political environment characterized by struggles between political parties over agenda setting and emphasis.

Conclusion and Discussion

The findings show how health agreement coordination became established by:

- Shared narratives of secure operations, letting the goals become administrative (not political), and making concrete delivery plans to ensure the agreements became a success, for the press and at the

National Board of Health, as they are important matters for creating legitimate relationships.

- Shared narratives of an equal partnership, as politicians build up trust in SKUs, allowing the committees to become a new governance steering tool and creating new meeting places for trustful dialogues between municipalities and regions, thus opening the door for pluricentric coordination with many centers of authority.
- Shared narratives of control, which became a way to handle political maneuvering for politicians by installing and controlling meeting agendas.

These elements demonstrate how shared narratives had different coordination impacts. The first narratives resulted in delivery plans and built on a design understanding of coordination, requiring a tight coupling between the health care providers. The second shared narratives created the condition of pluricentric coordination and are related to the first two, by sharing a need to make successful narratives. The narratives also demonstrated discoordination, or more loosely coupled relations, as the politicians moved the responsibility of work to the individual service providers. These narratives also took into account that coordination of the health care agreements can be understood as a medical issue, not well suited for political statements in the press, concerning local communities' growth and wellbeing as the main legitimate matters for politicians.

The first two narratives are epic narratives told as noble achievements, as indicated by the emotion and pride they include (Gabriel, 2000, p. 74; see Chapter 2). The last narrative was told as a tragedy, as an undeserved misfortune, with the emotion of fear or sorrow emerging (Gabriel, 2000, p. 70). The politicians and administrators talked about the loss of freedom and having to work under conditions of strict control, which did not allow them to express their ideas. They became victims of the meetings. Thus the three shared narratives were all structured narratives with a coherent succession of events leading to a plot (of achievement or of a loss of freedom).

When we moved our ethnographic studies from a focus on hospital wards to regional political centers, the organizational members and external stakeholders shifted. Health care professionals as well as the press became external stakeholders, and politicians and administrators became the organizational members. By doing ethnographic work, and following the different meetings, it became possible to conduct more informal interviews, during which both administrators and politicians talked about solutions as well as problems in the process.

Administrators' and politicians' daily work in meetings provides examples of everyday organizing in health care contexts, and their narratives and coordination negotiations impact the work in hospital wards.

In these examples, making concrete delivery plans and trying to forge a new culture of accepting the values of other service providers also created space for the local service providers to operate independently.

This chapter shared an example of how the political and administrative tasks of coordination also become an example of organizational change in a health care setting. Politicians and administrators were making sense of coordination in three shared narratives to create new coordination routines at the regional health care level. In contrast to the hospital ward level and everyday innovation, politically initiated change processes have their own life in meetings and become a part of everyday life and organizing for politicians and administrators. Patient values are not the main concern for these participants, as values concerning the press, the voter community, and telling success narratives were legitimately valued in these change processes.

Note

1. This presentation of coordination theories is part of a theoretical study that was conducted as part of a larger research project, "The Formation of a Region," steered by Professor Eva Sørensen and Karina Sehested. This research project also included the empirical data presented in the second part of the chapter. Some of the results are also published in the book: "Offentlig styring som pluricentrisk coordination. 2011, Ed. Sørensen et al., København. DJØF Forlag. and the article: "Emerging theoretical understanding of pluricentric coordination in public governance (2011). Both publications were written together with Eva Sørensen and Karina Sehested. The project was partly funded by the Danish VAT Foundation. I thank Eva Sørensen and Karina Sehested for lively and vibrant discussions and inspiration. The results of this research project are still relevant today, as renewed health agreements have become a major policy instruments used to enforce collaboration between municipalities and regions. Even if the policy areas shift in the new contracts (2019–2023), the basic development of the health agreements as administratively driven and as a partnership model remains the dominant value.

References

Borum, F. (2004). Means-end frames and the politics and myths of organizational fields. *Organization Studies, 25*(6), 897–921.

Czarniawska, B., & Joerges, B. C. (1997). *Narrating the organization: Dramas of institutional identity*. Chicago, IL: University of Chicago Press.

Fairhurst, G. T., & Putnam, L. (2004). Organizations as discursive constructions. *Communication Theory, 14*(1), 5–26.

Fayol, H. (1949). *General and industrial management*. London: Pitman.

Friedland, R., & Alford, R. R. (1991). Bringing society back in: Symbols, practices, and institutional contradictions. In W. W. Powell & P. J. DiMaggio (Eds.), *The new institutionalism in organizational analysis* (pp. 232–267). Chicago, IL: University of Chicago Press.

Gabriel, Y. (2000). *Storytelling in organizations: Facts, fictions and fantasies.* Oxford, UK: Oxford University Press.

Lindblom, C. E. (1959). The science of "muddling through". *Public Administration Review, 19*(2), 79–88.

March, J. G., & Olsen, J. P. (1989). *Rediscovering institutions: The organizational basis of politics.* New York, NY: The Free Press.

Meyer, J. W., & Rowan, B. (1977). Institutionalized organizations: Formal structure as myth and ceremony. *American Journal of Sociology, 83*(2), 340.

Mikkelsen, E. N., Petersen, A., & Pedersen, A. R. (2016). Problemer i det tværfaglige, tværorganisatoriske, tværsektorielle samarbejde i psykiatrien. *Tidsskrift for Arbejdsliv, 18*(3), 9–27.

Mintzberg, H. (1983). *Structure in fives: Designing effective organisations.* Upper Saddle River, NJ: Prentice Hall.

Mintzberg, H., & Westley, F. (1992). Cycles of organisational change. *Strategic Management Journal, 13*(S2), 39–59.

Orton, J. D., & Weick, K. E. (1990). Loosely coupled systems: A reconceptualization. *The Academy of Management Review, 15*(2), 203–223.

Pedersen, A. R., Sehested, K., & Sørensen, E. (2011). Emerging theoretical understanding of pluricentric coordination in public governance. *The American Review of Public Administration, 41*(4), 375–394.

Perrow, C. (1967). A framework for the comparative analysis of organizations. *American Sociological Review, 32*(2), 194–208.

Quinn, R. W., & Dutton, J. E. (2005). Coordination as energy-in-conversation. *The Academy of Management Review, 30*(1), 36–57.

Scott, W. R. (1987). *Organizations: Rational, natural, and open systems.* Upper Saddle River, NJ: Prentice Hall.

Sørensen, E., Sehested, K., & Pedersen, A. R. (2011). *Offentlig styring som pluricentrisk koordination.* København: Djøf Forlag.

Taylor, F. W. (1949). *The principles of scientific management.* Boston, MA: Adamant Media Corporation.

Thompson, J. D. (1967). *Organizations in action: Social science bases of administrative theory.* New York, NY: McGraw-Hill College.

Thornton, P. H., Ocasio, W., & Lounsbury, M. (2012). *The institutional logics perspective: A new approach to culture, structure, and process.* Oxford, UK: Oxford University Press on Demand.

Van de Ven, A. H., Delbecq, A. L., & Koenig, R. Jr. (1976). Determinants of coordination modes within organizations. *American Sociological Review, 41*(2), 322–338.

Waldorff, S. B., Reay, T., & Goodrick, E. (2013). A tale of two countries: How different constellations of logics impact action. In *Institutional logics in action, Part A* (pp. 99–129). Emerald Group Publishing Limited.

Weick, K. E. (1993). The collapse of sensemaking in organizations: The Mann Gulch Disaster. *Administrative Science Quarterly, 38*(4), 628–652.

7 Policy Narratives of Innovation Expectations

The purpose of this chapter is to demonstrate how organizational change and innovation in a health care setting also relates to the policy narratives. Policy narratives of innovations are policy instruments to guide the political expectations of how to become an innovative health care organization. The main assumption is that narratives of everyday innovation also address political values regarding policy innovation embedded in different public management ideas, as all narratives relate to other types of narratives. In this case, this chapter will explore how policy narratives of innovation relates to public management ideas.

Once every year, I meet with head doctors from the whole country to discuss the current conditions of management at hospitals with them. Public management perspectives are a part of these meetings that they really like, as they can all relate to the different public management perspectives because they are confronted with new steering methods on a yearly base. Lean meetings are currently being implemented at many clinical wards in one region, patient surveys are a national evaluation routine, and value-based care management is a new steering model many wards are implementing to change the finance model from activity-based to value-based steering. Many of these steering methods derive from public management perspectives. One sensemaking condition for organizational change processes is that they are in a field containing multiple public management ideas and therefore need to address multiple legitimate public management ideas and policy expectations.

Thus a policy condition for organizational change includes national policy papers addressing policy expectations for the development of health care organizations as innovative organizations in order to follow the general development in society and continue to remain legitimate health care organizations as approaches and policies evolve. Policy narratives are inspired by different sets of public management ideas over time. This means the criteria for legitimation of innovative hospital organizing is evolving as it connects to different public management assumptions and perspectives. This leaves innovative health care organizing in a dynamic steering context of sensemaking of different policy expectations.

In the first part of the chapter three public management perspectives, which have dominated the literature of public management in the last 20 years, will be presented, including traditional public administration, new public management, and network governance (Considine & Lewis, 2003; Ferlie, Lynn, & Pollitt, 2007; Pollitt, 2003). The first part will describe the central concepts and assumptions of these three public management perspectives.

The second part of the chapter will present three policy narratives as shared structured narratives from policy papers. These papers are about innovation in society and demonstrate the development of policy expectations over time. The three narratives also help to identify what the innovation problems are and how innovation solutions contain certain kinds of activities. The three policy narratives shared express an innovation journey, from understanding innovation as an activity primarily occurring in private organizations, to its becoming an important activity in public organizations.

The three policy narratives are findings from a document study of policy regulations over time. The aim of the study was to collect all relevant policy papers describing public innovation over time and to identify patterns in these papers. Using a qualitative data method, three shared narratives were found illustrating three different understandings of public service innovation over time.

The contribution of the chapter is to demonstrate how policy narratives of innovation relate to organizational narratives of everyday innovation, to demonstrate how multiple dominant values and meanings regarding innovation influence organizational change processes.

Theories of Public Management Perspectives

The three dominating public management perspectives presented include public administration (PA), new public management (NPM), and network governance (NG), in addition to each perspective's core concepts and assumptions for steering and organizing. The last part of this section brings all of the perspectives together in a table to detail the internal differences in the underlying principles of organizing, what actions the organizational members take, their legitimation, and the environment. The conclusion also brings in an example of a potential new public management perspective, pointing to the dynamic and continuous development of public management understandings and perspectives.

Public Administration

It would be difficult, today, to imagine the public sector without bureaucracy as its core organizational model. It is still an unquestionable approach in public sector management, and for many good reasons. Johan Olsen (2005) argues that for those interested in how contemporary public administration is organized, functions, and changes, it is worthwhile to reconsider and rediscover bureaucracy as an administrative form, an analytical concept, and a set of ideas and observations about public administration and formally organized institutions.

(p. 2)

So, even though bureaucracy has a long history, the ideas remain relevant today (Pedersen & Waldorff, 2019).

The public administration (PA) approach emerged during the postwar period in the course of the development of public sectors and welfare states. The political concern was to assure citizens' rights and access to public services. The PA approach builds upon bureaucracy as its core organizational model. Weber (1947, 1971) explained the rise of bureaucracy as a particular organizational form which provides the ground rules for organizing public service. In the bureaucratic approach, the power and authority lie with the government, and decisions are implemented top-down. There is a distinction between political and administrative decisions and a rational decision making chain in which some decisions have to do with policymaking, whereas others have to do with implementation (Diefenbach & Todnem, 2009; Olsen, 2005; Simon, 1950). Politicians are passionate and visionary policymakers, whereas the ethos of the public managers and employees is to be neutral and loyal when they carry out the policies (du Gay, 2000).

The organization is a hierarchy of distributed responsibilities and clear division of work, the practices are regulated through standards, rules and legislation, and the managerial focus is on employees' competences. This is to ensure that decisions and assessments of services for citizens are based upon a competent and legal-rational foundation. In this context, planning is important and defined as the programmed and strictly regulated distribution of tasks following specific rules (Perrow, 1967). The understanding is that the public sector should be managed by knowledge standardization but also accept a high degree of autonomy by the professionals working in them (Pedersen & Waldorff, 2019).

In this approach managerial tasks are concentrated on implementing policies through the creation of formal hierarchy and comprehensive administrative practices and procedures. The precondition is that public managers possess the professional knowledge and expertise relevant for implementing the policies in concrete practices, such as law regulation and public service, and also for ensuring the high professional quality of the organization's performance. The focus is on organizational input, such as hiring public managers with proper educational backgrounds and work experience into the organization. Some studies support this model, arguing that a bureaucratic organization does particularly well in implementation (Pierce and Delbecq, 1977). Paul du Gay (2000) argued further that bureaucracy—despite persistent critical discourse—is a suitable organizational model, which is capable of ensuring democratic control, quality, and continuity in a nation-state's performance, nationally and internationally (Pedersen & Waldorff, 2019).

In the bureaucratic approach, the attention to the external environment lies particularly with the politicians. It is the politicians' ideas that address societal challenges and developments and create political visions that public organizations are required to implement. This understanding, however, builds upon the notion that politicians and the public organizations together are capable of solving pressing and pending societal challenges. For many years this understanding seemed reasonable, but in recent years, the neo-Weberian approach stresses the relevance of a more responsive state (Pollitt & Bouckaert, 2011, p. 25ff). This means that the public sector needs to open up and listen to citizens' needs. Such organizations will still rely on the judgment of professionals, but the professionals should be much more aware of citizens' needs (Pedersen & Waldorff, 2019).

The public administration approach has also been criticized for its rigid standardization of procedures and also for prioritizing high professional quality in services over cost considerations and efficiency. Some have argued that this is due to professionals' focus on providing the best solutions for citizens, or, more critically, securing their own jobs and resources (Courpasson & Reed, 2004). However, in the neo-Weberian approach, there is an increased attention on efficiency. This means that managerial roles and tasks have changed, so it is important to combine high professional quality with cost utilization and efficiency (Pollitt & Bouckaert, 2011).

Summing up, from the 1950s and onward, strong belief in the advantages of bureaucratic forms were met by critical voices arguing that bureaucratic forms of rule tended to produce implementation resistance, silo thinking, and unintended consequences (Hull & Hjern, 1982; Pressman & Wildavsky, 1973; Simon, 1950).

New Public Management

The new public management (NPM) reforms of the 1980s and 1990s aimed to remedy the shortcomings of bureaucracy by introducing new forms of steering. NPM focuses on hands-on management, explicit standards and measures of organizational performance, greater emphasis on output control, disaggregation of units in the public sector, greater competition, emphasis on private sector styles of management practice, and stress on greater discipline and parsimony in resource use (Hood, 1991, p. 5).

Organizations practicing NPM should split up large public sector hierarchies and achieve wider, flatter ways of organizing. NPM also implies stronger flexibility and the inclusion of other supportive information systems (Dunleavy, Margetts, Bastow, & Tinkler, 2006). Disaggregation through the division of larger organizational units is one of the core elements of organizing in NPM. Making divisions between a provider and a purchaser is also part of this structure. The provider can be outsourced, so the main public part is the core area of the state administration of different providers. The underlying understanding in this perspective is that formal organizational structures are important. NPM's understanding of organizations builds on ideas from early studies of organizations that focused on single private organizations, which could be optimized by studies of work conditions, management rules, and workforce conditions. Scientific management studies were partly performed by managers and partly by researchers investigating the machinery of organizations (Taylor, 1949). They experimented with the management of work through different patterns of work divisions, standardization, and direct supervision. These studies laid the groundwork for organizational design studies. This view of the organizations is in line with other studies at that time focusing on single organizations, just shifted into the private sector. The inspiration and influence of the scientific management studies is visible in NPM thinking and the assumption that organizations can be designed in one best way to facilitate control and strong performance (Pedersen & Waldorff, 2019).

Hood (1995) described how NPM stressed two new management doctrines. One of these was to challenge the earlier distinct sharp line between the private sector and the public sector in regard to separate ways of doing business, having a distinct organizational design, rewards, and carrier structures. Instead, there were lessons to be learned from the private sector in the public sector. The second doctrinal shift was a greater emphasis in accountability in terms of results rather than processes (p. 94). These two management lines resulted in hands-on management approaches, with the underlying assumption that decentralized and strong local leadership with inspiration from the private sector would also be relevant in the public sector. Given the professional knowledge and the tradition of public professionals, the transition to becoming managers without managerial skills was a challenge. The bureaucratic distinction between politics and administration is not the challenges, but a third dimension is added into the formal management line: politicians, administrators, and managers. Management is seen as applying rational processes that can be planned and designed in different steps; beginning with an urgent platform and ending with institutionalization (Fernandez & Rainey, 2006). The new responsibility of public managers is to manage and lead public organization as effective organizations, but at a distance from politicians and political decisions. NPM means that the public sector should implement management principles and models from the private sector, such as agency-provider structures, total quality management, and LEAN. An examination of public and private organizations showed that they increasingly exhibited the same management approaches, with inspiration from Kotter (1995), among others (Pedersen & Waldorff, 2019).

Some of the main foundational considerations of NPM are the market and competition. The competition is linked to pecuniary-based performance incentives, with inspiration from principle and agent theory from economics, or public service motivation theory (Laffont & Martimort, 2009; Perry, 2000).

The paradigm of NPM created massive regulatory reforms, tried to ensure market competition between public and private organizations and outsourcing, and focused on ensuring change through targets, goals, and policy effects. This also included increased output control, introducing process evaluations, standards, quality measurements, and output evaluations. This development started in the UK but spread widely to other European countries, starting as a political movement and becoming an administrative reform wave with a broad focus on output control and user satisfaction in all public organizations. The inspiration also came from organizational behavior, with a focus on individual, group, and organizational system behavior (Robbins, Judge & Campbell, 2010).

Summing up, NPM built on classical bureaucratic organizational assumptions of formal structures and work division combined with rational step-by-step designed leadership theory and incentives and organizational behavior theory. This cluster of different organizational understandings characterizes NPM as a diverse steering perspective, with many internal conflicts. These findings appear paradoxical, and one of the consequences is the tensions between the three underlying principles of NPM (Ferlie, 1996) and the recent studies illustrating the unseen consequences of NPM ways of organizing (Diefenbach, 2009).

Network Governance

Network governance (NG) is a public management approach that came after NPM and is often presented as a critique of NPM. NG researchers criticize the assumption shared by the traditional theories of PA and NPM, thinking that public management can be obtained without persistent interaction and communication between the involved and affected parties in the decision chain. Governance theorists argue that the level of complexity, diversity, and dynamism of the problems and issues that confront public governors highlights the need for a theoretical reframing of PA research (Kickert, Klijn, & Koppenjan, 1997; Kooiman, 2003; Rhodes, 1997). NG is not a narrow approach but rather a common description for many public network approaches that share an understanding of public organizations as networks, and therefore it breaks with past understandings of organizations, management, and change processes. The network approaches share a belief and interest in relatively stable and interdependent autonomous actors, interacting through negotiations that contribute to the production of public purpose (Sørensen & Torfing, 2006).

Governance can be studied as a disordered and complex process in which a plurality of public and private actors, including politicians and public administrators, interact in more or less formalized negotiation processes that lead to the authorization and implementation of political decisions. These forms of interactive collaboration, and in particular governance networks, were inspired by the theoretical concept of mutual dependency (Sørensen & Torfing, 2006, p. 9). Several different theories endeavor to explain the patterns of networks and interaction, moving from formal and individualist calculation to descriptive mapping of networks. They share a common interest of looking at policy problems instead of policy solutions, and the wicked problem theory has been one form of argumentation regarding how to understand policy processes by defining complex policy problems (Head & Alford, 2015). Central network concepts in many governance theories include trust, communication, interaction, and negotiations, along with enhancing the inter-professional, inter-organizational, and inter-departmental relations. Some network studies are inspired by organizational design, borrowing from its emphasis on guiding, functions, and interest among the stakeholders, wherein networks can be designed and facilitated in different directions to address specific policy problems (Kickert et al., 1997; Klijn & Koppenjan, 2004). Others make a distinction between policy networks and governance networks, and between interpretative and decentered networks, incorporating social network analysis—the latter being more quantitative than the former (Lewis, 2011; Pedersen & Waldorff, 2019).

Because network autonomy is incompatible with traditional forms of ensuring public management (Byrkjeflot & du Gay, 2012), governance theorists claim that interactive forms of NG call for a new form of management that allows for designed and facilitated networks as well as self-steering or meta-governance (Sørensen, 2006). Meta-governance emphasizes the various mechanisms that public authority and other resourceful actors can use to initiate and stimulate negotiated self-governance among relevant stakeholders and/or guide them in a certain direction (Sørensen, 2006).

Summing up, governance is seen as a complex process in which a plurality of public and private actors interact in more or less formalized negotiation processes that lead to the implementation of political decisions. These forms of interactive collaboration, and in particular governance networks, were theoretically inspired by the concept of mutual dependency (Sørensen & Torfing, 2006, p. 9).

Partial Discussion and Conclusion

Public management theories affect the societal understanding of steering and organizing principles, such as the roles of organizations, organizational members, users, and environments. For example, in PA, patients are understood as democratic citizens and receivers of services, but with the introduction of NPM a new role expectation of patients emerged, wherein patients were now perceived as customers or users. In an opposite perspective, the NG perspective defines patients as co-creators and partners in collaborative networks. All of these role expectations are sensemaking conditions of how to understand patients in hospitals through a new understanding in a dynamic policy context.

Table 7.1 presents the different core concepts and role expectations from the three different public management perspectives.

The table illustrates how PA depends on bureaucracy and the elements of hierarchy and knowledge. In PA, organizational members and managers have roles in relation to authority and expertise. The environment is the politicians as policymakers. The NPM perspective is organized through competition, markets, and efficiency, and the role of organizational members and managers is defined by individual performance. The last perspective, NG, is organized through network, relations, and partnerships, and the organizational members and managers are defined as co-creators and trustworthy and interactive communicators. This table summarizes the complex picture of how approaches to public organizing are theoretically defined and organized by different motivating principles, with different role expectations for members, users, and managers.

The three public management perspectives are not the only ones being debated in strands of public management. Public value is also a more recently developed public management approach (Moore, 2000; O'Flynn, 2007). The term was originally coined by Moore (1995), who

Table 7.1 Public Management Perspectives

	PA	NPM	NG
PERSPECTIVE	Bureaucracy	Competition	Networks
ORGANIZING PRINCIPLE	Hierarchy	Goal setting and strategies	Relations
MANAGER	Authority	Performance	Communication
CITIZEN	Passive receivers	Consumers	Co-creators
ORGANIZATIONAL MEMBER	Expertise and knowledge	Reacting on goals, work efficiency	Trust, communication, and interaction
LEGITIMACY/ AUTHORITY	Knowledge	Efficiency	Interdependency
ENVIRONMENT	Politicians	Markets	Partnerships

emphasized that the public sector is capable of creating a particular type of value—public value—which is equivalent to shareholder value in the private sector. Public value is a public organization's contribution to the common good and society, such as societal coherence, sustainability, or economic wealth. The background for this interest is a concern with complex societal problems for which there are no simple solutions, and from which global economic, ecological, politico-economic, technological, and social challenges create a complex context for public services (Benington & Moore, 2010; Pedersen & Waldorff, 2019).

Part 1 of this chapter demonstrated a picture of different public management perspectives, with internal contradictions and paradoxes but that, together, illustrate the dynamic policy steering context in which hospitals have to maneuver.

Shared Policy Narratives About Change and Innovation: From Knowledge Infrastructure to Welfare Improvements

The purpose of this second section is to demonstrate how shared policy narratives of public innovation develop over time and relate to multiple public management perspectives.

The findings were derived from a document study of a specific policy context, the empirical data was collected through a historical document analysis of public innovation policies in Denmark from 1999 to 2012. The data collection process initially began with the collection of policy documents to identify the policy narratives. First, we identified the private and public (state, regional, and local) organizations that we assumed would be relevant with regard to the production of policy documents that involved the concept of innovation. We then contacted these organizations to obtain their assistance in identifying additional policy actors and policy documents that would be particularly relevant for framing the policy approaches to public innovation in Denmark. We used this snowball technique, continuing the collection of data until no new sources for policy documents arose. Combined, we collected about 60 policy documents involving innovation published between 1999 and 2012. The earliest document that uses the word innovation was an annual report published by the Danish Ministry of Finance in 1999. Most of the documents collected were published from 2007 and on. We used a thematic analysis and NVivo software to analyze the data and identify the policy narratives. The policy narratives were systematically defined and categorized as we identified episodes that comprised problems, solutions, and stakeholder descriptions (Waldorff & Pedersen, 2013). A policy narrative became dominant when many policy documents described the policy problem and/or solution in the same manner. The narratives identified were thus formed as shared and structured narratives (Chapter 2). Three dominant policy narratives emerged from the analysis: the first was knowledge production innovation, which represents the early understanding of public innovation; the second is partnership innovation; and, finally, public welfare innovation describes the latest policy narrative.[1]

The First Narrative: Knowledge Production Innovation

The first policy narrative emerged in the early policy documents in 1999 and concerned the conditions for creating innovation in society. The policy narrative identified the problem as the creation of competitive advantages of private companies. This is emphasized in the following quote: "Efficient competition and well-functioning markets are essential conditions for a dynamic industry in which companies focus on development and innovation. Efficient competition forces companies to utilize resources and to constantly improve and develop products and manufacturing methods" (Danish finances, 2004).

The participants involved in this problem statement are private companies and public researchers, as this quotation shows: "The framework conditions of innovation consist of five main groups: public research, collaboration between research and private companies, innovation finance, collaboration with customers, competitors and suppliers and, last, access to competences and technology."

(A benchmark study of innovation and innovation policy:
What Denmark can learn, 2003, p. 2)

This document points to a list of the key actors of innovation: private companies, customers, competitors, and suppliers, all originating in the private sector. This is a dominant understanding of the most relevant actors that advocated for the advancement of innovation in society in the early development of innovation policy. During this time, innovation was understood as a phenomenon that flowered only in the private sector. The only public organizations mentioned are public research organizations that deliver knowledge to private companies, based on the premise that research and knowledge can lead to innovation (Waldorff & Pedersen, 2013).

Thus, knowledge is seen as the solution for securing national product development, and innovation is understood as a knowledge producing process involving public research organizations and private firms that will result in product development. The next policy document describes how utilizing knowledge is the solution to challenges in the market:

> Research alone does not create innovation. The knowledge generated by research institutions must be disseminated to businesses and used to develop new products and services. The business community's capacity to innovate depends on whether companies have good conditions for gaining knowledge and the right skills to use it. This requires an efficient infrastructure that supports the entire process from idea to discovering an application in a company. As a result, significantly more public resources must be spent to create the right environment for innovation in a broader sense.
>
> (Innovation at every level, 2005, p. 2)

A quote from another policy document from 2003 indicates how research-driven innovation was benefitting private companies:

> If public research is going to benefit the business community's research-driven innovation, then the interaction between the business community and public research, decisions concerning the direction of public research, and the conditions for interaction with the business community and public research are thus an important framework for research-driven innovation.
>
> (Three types of innovation, 2004, p. 5)

In this instance, knowledge production becomes the main plot of the policy narrative, describing how innovation is created when services or products are developed. This is in line with ideas of the market. Economic growth is a means to increase society's wealth. Innovation becomes a knowledge-based process, which includes research and private companies, and the actors in innovation are private companies, their ideas, and the opportunities they have available for using technology. The public organizations, e.g., research institutions, become an infrastructure that can add to and support, but not drive, innovation. The state idea is less profound in this narrative but is mobilized to legitimize the notion that economic growth is a means to improve the common good. The narrative constructs public knowledge production as the innovative solution. This policy narrative was dominant in many of the policy documents from 1999 and later (Waldorff & Pedersen, 2013).

The Second Narrative: Partnership Innovation

The second policy narrative emerged in 2005 and problematizes globalization as a threat to the national economy, and particularly the lack of resources and capabilities. This problem calls for formal structures with regard to many public areas, including health care, as the following indicates:

> Private stakeholders want greater cooperation with the public sector regarding health prevention efforts. They would like a forum for public-private organizations, and a place where social innovation can occur is the volunteer community where people are passionate about what they do. Providing more resources in this area creates a breeding ground for cooperation between local sports clubs and workplaces.
>
> (User health care: A proposal for patient reform in 2007, p. 3)

Thus, in the partnership' narrative, the governmental task is to leverage all possible societal resources to create innovation and new developments (Waldorff & Pedersen, 2013). The solution is to establish formal partnerships and networks and create close collaboration between private (including voluntary) and public organizations to foster innovation initiatives:

> The Innovation Council's goal is to be a catalyst for the renewal that Denmark must demonstrate, a task that the council cannot carry out alone, but we see the council as an important integral part of the innovation structure that society must develop in order to ensure the broad involvement of all the necessary resources. Simply put, this structure involves both a policy and a private aspect. The Danish

parliament must establish the policy and ensure the best conditions possible to develop the nation's capabilities.

(Innovation Council, 2005, p. 10)

This event also shows that the policy narrative mobilizes both market and state ideas, as it calls for a broad involvement of more types of resources and knowledge, including not only private companies but also politics, in the development of society. The underlying idea is that welfare derives from interaction based on market mechanisms but guided by policy and national regulation (Waldorff & Pedersen, 2013). The next statement shows how interdisciplinary work and diversity are important drivers of innovation:

> Interdisciplinarity and diversity give rise to new thinking and innovation. As a result, guaranteeing cooperation and synergy across sectors is an important aspect of research, development and innovation. This is the case not only for the vital interaction between knowledge environments and businesses, but also in the interaction between different disciplines—between the seller and the sociologist, the engineer, anthropologist and architect, and the machinist and the designer.
>
> (Increased knowledge transfer and innovation in the public sector, 2007, p. 5)

This quotation from a policy document describes a strong conviction toward collaboration across professions and sectors as a valuable aspect of sparking innovation and new ideas (Waldorff & Pedersen, 2013). Another quotation shows how the collaboration will also create better solutions and products:

> The employees and managers in public organizations do not always have all of the knowledge and skills necessary to develop welfare services. As a result, it is necessary to work with other players to develop these services. One example of a possible major partner is private companies or other public authorities with relevant knowledge that can be used in the development of new solutions and products that the public sector demands.
>
> (Growth and prosperity: Catalogue of Recommendations, 2011, p. 4)

The second policy narrative thus differed from the first one by pointing out that the problem is the lack of resources at the national level (Waldorff & Pedersen, 2013). Partnerships are then considered to be the innovative solution to this problem, and new public organizations were emerging as aggregators of such partnerships.

The Last Narrative: Public Welfare Innovation

The last policy narrative we identified in the policy documents emphasized the problem of the public sector's lack of capability to solve complex societal problems, such as obesity, environmental pollution, and juvenile delinquency. The task was to overcome this public sector inertia. Thus, this last policy narrative described innovation as a process that occurs within public sector organizations that can lead to reforms and equip the organizations to better solve future welfare and public service issues. Attention moved from innovation as an activity of the private sector to a public sector activity, which meant that the type of innovation also changed, from product- and user-driven innovation, to welfare and employee-driven innovation (Waldorff & Pedersen, 2013). This is reflected in this statement:

> The public sector also has to become more innovative. Future welfare challenges can only be solved in the coming decades if completely new ways of producing and delivering welfare services are developed.
> (Intelligent demand and public innovation proposals, 2010, p. 1)

In this quote, innovation is described as a solution to improve welfare. The narrative is legitimized by the democratic participation of more actors:

> Welfare innovation and technology focus on the innovations where employees work closely with citizens on solving daily welfare tasks. Welfare innovation is the ability to turn new ideas into values by improving workflow and introducing new technology, and this can happen in every public sector welfare area.
> (Public sector growth and welfare, 2011, p. 5)

This excerpt was different from the first policy narrative, where the main actors were from the private sector. Here, the mentioned actors are from public organizations, an indication that the driving actors in innovation processes are shifting from private to public actors. This means that public employees working in the public sector were now considered drivers of innovation, able to develop new solutions to complex problems and to improve efficiency and quality in service provision (Waldorff & Pedersen, 2013). The last policy narrative problematizes the public sector inertia and its capability to solve complex societal problems. Welfare innovation is constructed as the solution, stressing the important role of public employees. In this narrative, the individual employees need to assume the responsibility of creating innovative public organizations to deliver welfare in new and smarter ways.

Discussion and Conclusion

If we compare these three policy narratives, we can draw a picture to see how the first policy narrative is inspired by all of the public management perspectives. The main inspiration is thus, from NPM, from the perspective that competition is addressed as the main problem. The solution is to innovate new products by supporting new relations between the public research infrastructure and private companies. Innovation was seen as a domain of private companies and not for public organizations. They should deliver knowledge, whereas the private companies increase their market advantages. The second policy narrative changed the understanding and need for innovation, as globalization became a major political concern. The solutions are new partnerships, and as such, this policy narrative strongly draws on ideas from NG. But the partnership should be managed partly by public support and policies and by strong partnership leaderships. Thereby other public management perspectives are also implied in this narration. The last policy narrative of innovation redirects the need for innovation in society to address complex societal problems, a dominating policy problem understanding from network and governance theories (Head & Alford, 2015). The solution is a need and focus on public organizations, which are now also recognized as places for innovation. Through new relations with users and citizens, welfare organizations should have a new capability to become innovative, also by enhancing the individual public employees' innovation skills. The third policy narratives not only draw on governance theory but also address the need for new technology, product development, and a strong belief in decentralized levels, which is also an inspiration from NPM thinking. In sum, it became difficult to compare distinct public management perspectives directly with the different policy narratives, but it's clear that the policy narratives drew inspiration from the three public management perspectives in different ways. Mixing ideas of competition, networks, incentives, trust, and user and policy steering draws a complex picture of the policy expectations that the policy narratives express regarding how to understand and make sense of innovation and the roles of public and private organizations in becoming more innovative.

The table illustrates the innovation problem, solution, stakeholder, and public management perspectives of the three policy narratives. Although they draw on different public management perspectives, the understandings of problems and solutions are foundationally inspired by different public management ideas, moving away from NPM and toward a network orientation. Yet the partnership and network developing does not address trust and communication as part of network building (Torfing & Sørensen, 2006), but it addresses the steering of ideas from both PA and NPM thinking (innovation policies and stronger local management).

Table 7.2 Policy Narratives and Public Management Perspectives

Policy narratives	Knowledge production	Partnerships	Employee and user innovation
INNOVATION PROBLEM	Competition	Globalization	Complex social problems
INNOVATION SOLUTIONS	Efficient competition, new products	Partnerships	Innovative public organizations
STAKEHOLDERS	Private companies and public research	Mix of sectors, new aggregators	Users and public employees
PUBLIC ADMINISTRATION ORIENTATION	Public research structure	Public partnership infrastructure	Employee driven innovation
NEW PUBLIC MANAGEMENT ORIENTATION	Market orientation	Contracts/ partnerships	Development of new technologies
GOVERNANCE ORIENTATION	New relations between public and private	Inter-disciplinarity Diversity	Collaboration with citizens

This chapter contributes to an understanding of a dynamic policy context for health care organizations as policy narratives evolve over time, expressing multiple policy expectations toward how to be innovative. The policy expectations in the policy narratives are inspired by different and contradictory public management perspectives, which leaves health care change management in a complex and dynamic policy context. The right political way to become innovative hospitals is to build up the knowledge and research infrastructure, to enter into partnerships with private and voluntary organizations, and to foster innovative employees who are able to interact with users to gain new perspectives on potential innovative solutions. The last policy narrative supports the local professional values of patient involvement, which was also demonstrated in Chapter 5. Together, these findings address policy conditions of organizational change processes in specific policy contexts. They also demonstrate how shared policy narratives developed over time and created legitimate sensemaking regarding the approaches and processes of supporting innovation.

Note

1. These results can also be found in Waldorff, S. B., & Pedersen, A. R. (2013). Hybridization of institutional logics and narrative accounts in policy

documents. *EGOS Paper.* I thank Susanne Boch Waldoff for an ongoing inspiring research collaboration.

References

Benington, J., & Moore, M. H. (Eds.). (2010). *Public value: Theory and practice.* Macmillan International Higher Education.

Byrkjeflot, H., & du Gay, P. (2012). Bureaucracy: An idea whose time has come (again)? In T. Diefenbach & R. Todnem (Eds.), *Reinventing hierarchy and bureaucracy: From the bureau to network organizations* (pp. 85–109). Bingley, UK: Emerald Group Publishing Limited.

Considine, M., & Lewis, J. M. (2003). Bureaucracy, network, or enterprise? Comparing models of governance in Australia, Britain, the Netherlands, and New Zealand. *Public Administration Review, 63*(2), 131–140.

Courpasson, D., & Reed, M. (2004). Introduction: Bureaucracy in the age of enterprise. *Organization, 11*(1), 5–12.

Diefenbach, T. (2009). New public management in public sector organizations: The dark sides of managerialistic "enlightenment". *Public Administration, 87*(4), 892–909.

Diefenbach, T., & Todnem, R. (2009). Reinventing hierarchy and bureaucracy: From the bureau to network organizations. In M. Lounsbury (Ed.), *Research in the sociology of organizations* (Vol. 35). Bingley, UK: Emerald Group Publishing Limited.

Du Gay, P. (2000). *In praise of bureaucracy: Weber, organization, ethics.* London: Sage.

Dunleavy, P., Margetts, H., Bastow, S., & Tinkler, J. (2006). New public management is dead-long live digital-era governance. *Journal of Public Administration Research and Theory, 16*(3), 467–494.

Ferlie, E. (1996). *The new public management in action.* New York, NY: Oxford University Press.

Ferlie, E., Lynn, L. E., & Pollitt, C. (2007). *The Oxford handbook of public management.* New York, NY: Oxford University Press.

Fernandez, S., & Rainey, H. G. (2006). Managing successful organizational change in the public sector. *Public Administration Review,* March-April, 168–176.

Head, B. W., & Alford, J. (2015). Wicked problems: Implications for public policy and management. *Administration & Society, 47*(6), 711–739.

Hood, C. (1991). A new public management for all seasons. *Public Administration, 69*(1), 1–19.

Hood, C. (1995). The "new public management" in the 1980s: Variations on a theme. *Accounting, Organizations and Society, 20*(2), 93–109.

Hull, C., & Hjern, B. (1982). Helping small firms grow: An implementation analysis of small firm assistance structures. *European Journal of Political Research, 10*(2), 187–198.

Kickert, W. J., Klijn, E. H., & Koppenjan, J. F. (Eds.). (1997). *Managing complex networks: Strategies for the public sector.* London: Sage.

Klijn, E.-H., & Koppenjan, J. (2004). *Managing uncertainties in networks.* London: Routledge.

Kooiman, J. (2003). *Governing as governance*. London: Sage.

Kotter, J. P. (1995). Leading change: Why transformation efforts fail. *Harvard Business Review, 73*, 59–67.

Laffont, J. J., & Martimort, D. (2009). *The theory of incentives: The principal-agent model*. Princeton, NJ: Princeton University Press.

Lewis, J. M. (2011). The future of network governance research: Strength in diversity and synthesis. *Public Administration, 89*(4), 1221–1234.

Moore, M. (1995). *Creating public value: Strategic management in government*. Cambridge, MA: Harvard University Press.

Moore, M. H. (2000). Managing for value: Organizational strategy in for-profit, nonprofit and governmental organizations. *Nonprofit and Voluntary Sector Quarterly, 29*(1), 183–204.

O'Flynn, J. (2007). From new public management to public value: Paradigmatic change and managerial implications. *Australian Journal of Public Administration, 66*(3), 353–366.

Olsen, J. P. (2005). Maybe it is time to rediscover bureaucracy. *Journal of Public Administration Research and Theory, 16*(1), 1–24.

Pedersen, A. R., & Waldorff, B. S. (2019). Public management approaches addressing organizational elements towards situational public management. *IRSPM Conference Paper*, Wellington.

Perrow, C. (1967). A framework for the comparative analysis of organizations. *American Sociological Review, 32*(2), 194–208.

Perry, J. L. (2000). Bringing society in: Toward a theory of public-service motivation. *Journal of Public Administration Research and Theory, 10*(2), 471–488.

Pierce, J. L., & Delbecq, A. L. (1977). Organization structure, individual attitudes and innovation. *Academy of Management Review, 2*(1), 27–37.

Pollitt, C. (2003). *The essential public manager*. London: McGraw-Hill Education.

Pollitt, C., & Bouckaert, G. (2011). *Public management reform: A comparative analysis-new public management, governance, and the Neo-Weberian state*. Oxford, UK: Oxford University Press.

Pressman, J. L., & Wildavsky, A. (1973). *Implementation*. Berkeley: University of California Press.

Rhodes, R. A. W. (1997). *Understanding governance: Policy networks, governance, reflexivity and accountability*. Buckingham: Open University Press.

Robbins, S. P., Judge, T., & Campbell, T. (2010). *Organizational behavior*. London: Pearson Education.

Simon, H. (1950). Administrative behaviour. *Australian Journal of Public Administration, 9*(1), 241–245.

Sørensen, E. (2006). Metagovernance: The changing role of politicians in processes of democratic governance. *The American Review of Public Administration, 36*(1), 79–97.

Sørensen, E., & Torfing, J. (Eds.). (2006). *Theories of democratic network governance*. London: Palgrave Macmillan.

Taylor, F. W. (1949). *The principles of scientific management*. Boston, MA: Adamant Media Corporation.

Waldorff, S. B., & Pedersen, A. R. (2013). Hybridization of institutional logics and narrative accounts in policy documents. *EGOS Paper*, Montreal.

Weber, M. (1947). *The theory of social and economic organization*. London: Collier Macmillan Publishers.
Weber, M. (1971). *Makt og byråkrati*. Oslo: Gyldendals Norsk Forlag.
Weber, M., Lassman, P., Velody, I., & Martins, H. (1989). *Max Weber's "science as a vocation"*. London: Unwin & Hyman.

White papers from Danish ministries:

Department of Finance. (2004). "Danish finances".
Department of Finance. (2011). "Growth and prosperity: Catalogue of Recommendations", 1.
Department of Modernization. (2003). "A benchmark study of innovation and innovation policy: What Denmark can learn".
Department of Modernization. (2004). "Three types of innovation".
Department of Modernization. (2005). "Innovation at every level".
Department of Modernization. (2010). "Intelligent demand and public innovation proposals".
Department of Modernization. (2011). "Public sector growth and welfare".
Innovation Council. (2005). "Innovation Council Annual Report: Innovative Denmark".
Innovation Council. (2007). "Increased knowledge transfer and innovation in the public sector".
The Ministry of Health. (2007). "User health care: A proposal for patient reform".

8   Concluding Remarks

The intention of this conclusion is to answer the research questions presented in the first chapter of the book, which were:

> *How can we understand organizational change by doing an everyday ethnography?*
> *Which narratives can be found when making sense of organizational change processes?*
> *In addition, what are the sensemaking consequences for organizational change processes?*

These research questions can be answered by presenting three different results. The first question is related to the used of ethnography as a qualitative field method, and how this method and research focus added insight into a micro-context, in contrast to Van de Ven, Polley, Garud, and Venkatarman's (1999) macro-oriented context understanding. The second question refers to the kinds of narratives that can be found in ethnographic studies. The third and last question refers to the kinds of sensemaking that were identified.

Observing and Interacting With and From the Front

> *How can we understand organizational change by doing everyday ethnography?*

In Chapter 2, organizational change was defined as ongoing continuous processes of change, meaning that change is a part of everyday organizing. One argument in organizational ethnographic studies is that the method of doing ethnography should have an influence on how we define the phenomena under study. Often, ethnographic studies do not connect their findings to the methods they used, or treat the organization as a place to conduct field studies (Pedersen & Humle, 2016). Undertaking an everyday ethnography has implications for how organizational change in an everyday context can be understood.

When conducting field studies in health care organizations, one observes these organizations as places where people meet. An ethnographic approach cannot provide a full picture of all of the interactions (Ybema, Yanow, Wels, & Kamsteeg, 2009); however, an everyday ethnography can demonstrate how daily interactions and narratives are part of making sense of organizational change.

In hospital settings, the daily workers are health care professionals and clinical managers, who are present every day. Patients come and go in endless streams, as well as external stakeholders, including consultants, representatives from patient associations, and visiting administrators from public authorities. Not on a daily basis, but often, in a regional setting, politicians and administrators also come and go in endless streams, along with citizens, external health care professionals, and other external stakeholders occasionally visiting. Health care organizations are not closed entities; they are living organizations, formed by patients' and health care professionals' interactions, politicians' and administrators' policy goals, and collaborations that involve many different stakeholders, all making sense of what is going on by voicing narratives.

Some narratives relate to policy narratives, as they are told in a web of communication and expression. Such narratives are not final products but unfold in the process of negotiating and relating to other narratives. To collect organizational narratives (Gabriel, 2000) means listening and talking with people in the organizations on a daily basis. Narratives analyzed from interviews and field observations can be described as backstage narratives when they are being told about work routines in work scenes in waiting rooms and in offices. One can discover the daily interactions and collaborations between both internal and external organizational members, and the many ways in which shared narratives of participation emerge; however, resistance and struggles are a common aspect of narratives. Both shared and more fragmented sensemaking are found in the narratives.

What becomes of organizational change, then? We have seen how change emerges as newly established routines in an emergency ward and how resistance to or support for organizational change is related to the values of health care professionals. We have identified strong shared values regarding patient ownership and additional values associated with waiting time and meetings when coordinating with each other. Organizational change is not an impossible quest. Two local collaborative innovation projects demonstrated how values of patient involvement and shared meanings of engagement and materialization led to new ways of conducting a medical interview and treatment of patients waiting at the wards. But the local values of health care professionals are not the only condition of organizational change and innovation in everyday contexts. Narratives about how to make secured operations, equal partnerships, and control can also facilitate administrative regional coordination of the activities of different health care providers and organizations, including hospitals. Coordination of activities involves developing detailed delivery plans to address certain work routines such as discharge processes. As highlighted by the National Board of Health, health professionals are an integral part of organizational change processes, as they address the top-down issues that wards are involved in by participating in ad hoc committees. The identified coordination problems were formulated as administrative and political agendas, a long way from the clinical wards, but they demonstrate how new change items also are often introduced.

A final result of understanding organizational change through ethnographic study is the variety of different types of change narratives illustrating national policy narratives that described participants' expectations toward innovation. Three policy narratives defined various innovation challenges, including competition, globalization, and solving complex societal problems, as well as addressing assorted possibilities: research structure, partnerships, and the value of innovative employees and user input. The last policy narratives supported the values of patient empowerment. These values were also visible in the innovation design projects presented in Chapter 5, stressing the possible connections and disconnections between policy narratives of innovation and local organizational narratives of innovation.

Organizational change has many faces. New emerging routines at local wards, with a focus on prioritizing patients, talking about and understanding the diagnosis processes, and improving wait times. There are also the administrative tasks of crafting delivery plans to coordinate between health care providers and policy expectations for becoming innovative. These are all mundane change ambitions, but from a frontline worker's perspective, what is more important than prioritizing patients, giving them their (cancer) diagnosis in the best way, improving waiting conditions, and coordinating treatment between providers? Patients spend most of their time in hospitals waiting. Therefore, is a change project concerning their waiting time a small change project or a majorly important change project? All of the examples of organizational change that emerged in the process of doing everyday ethnographies are examples of frontline change processes, enhancing the importance of understanding change from frontline and everyday contexts (including several frontlines in hospitals and regions), where change projects most need to be made sense of by the participants.

Finding Individual and Collective Narratives

> *Which narratives can be found when making sense of organizational change processes?*

Organizational narratives are social constructions that illustrate how it is possible to persuade others and make shared sense of change ideas but also to clarify the unseen consequences and individual negative experiences of organizing change processes. The function of the organizational narratives in a health care setting is to illustrate organizational change processes as part of everyday organizing, including patients reflecting on their illness trajectories, the good intentions of clinical managers introducing evidence-based visitation routines, and health care professionals working to balance the implementation of new routines with patient needs, work conditions, and their own professional values and priorities. Everyday organizing is also challenged by local innovation projects, wherein the participants collaborate with design thinking devices to provoke their taken-for-granted knowledge, and detailed delivery plans are created between equal health care providers with the influence of policy expectations. Narratives create sensemaking conditions for coordination and innovation as distinct means of framing the needs of organizational change.

Table 8.1 lists the change studies, narratives, and sensemaking conditions to provide an overview of the previous section.

Fifteen different narratives from four ethnographic studies were presented. Of course, many more narratives were collected and identified in the studies, but 15 were selected to demonstrate the variety of narratives that contributed to sensemaking in change processes; some were individual narratives, others were shared.

Individual Narratives

In the analysis of the everyday change process in an ER triage, three individual narratives from a clinical manager, a patient, and health care professionals were presented.

The clinical manager shared a structured and strategic spokesperson narrative of the good intentions of the introduction of the triage model at the ward. The plot of his narrative described victories, struggles, and recognition in the narrative of the goal to persuade health care professionals to recognize that triage created faster and safer treatment for patients, and therefore it was a good idea. Thus, this narrative is shaped like an epic narrative (Gabriel, 2000).

The patient narrative was a structured tragic narrative of undeserved misfortune (Gabriel, 2000) in which the patient talked about being invalidated subjugated by the needs of acute patients. She had to wait a long time, was starving, and felt sorry for herself, not to mention afraid of not getting results. She shared an individual illness narrative of patient values wherein waiting time, hygiene, food, and transportation matters.

The various ante-narratives of health care professionals were about ambiguity and tensions (Pedersen & Humle, 2016) as part of understanding the new triage activities. The health care professionals talked about ambiguity in ante-narratives of new visible workloads, social control,

Table 8.1 Narratives and Sensemaking in Change Processes

	Narratives	*Sensemaking*
CHANGE AS EVERYDAY ORGANIZING IN A CLINICAL WARD	Individual narratives of: 1. Clinical manager 2. Patient 3. Health care professionals	Fragmented sensemaking: from the great change idea, to the terrible or unseen consequences
PROFESSIONALS' RESISTANCE TO CHANGE DUE TO EVERYDAY VALUES	Individual narratives of: 4. Professionals about patients 5. Professionals about other professionals	Sensemaking reflecting local values: patient autonomy interactions (battles)
DRIVERS FOR CHANGE WITH COLLABORATIVE PARTICIPANTS USING INNOVATIVE DESIGN	Shared/individual narratives: 6. Engagement 7. Materialization 8. Patients on waiting time 9. Participants on values	Shared sensemaking of the need for participation and individual sensemaking about the problems and solutions of the change projects
CHANGE AS THE NEED FOR COORDINATION BETWEEN HEALTH CARE PROVIDERS	Shared narratives: 10. Secure operations 11. Equal partnership 12. Control	Shared sensemaking becomes coordination, leading to coordination of activities
CHANGE AND INNOVATION EXPECTATIONS IN INNOVATION POLICIES	Shared narratives: 13. Knowledge production 14. Partnership 15. Welfare state innovation	Sensemaking in policy expectations and assumed sources of innovation

standardization of work tasks, and unethical conversations, which represented the unseen consequences of implementing the idea.

Together, these structured and fragmented individual narratives demonstrate how difficult it is to form an atmosphere of shared understanding in a change process, even if many agree that it is a good idea. Somebody will be the losers of the new system: from the patient not experiencing faster patient flows to the health care professionals experiencing new workloads and new social control. So, although the new triage model was presented as a good idea, the implementation had unseen organizing consequences, highlighting how change is intertwined with everyday organizing.

In the second analysis of the work of health care professionals at the rehabilitation ward, two types of individual narratives arose from the professionals about their collaboration with patients and colleagues.

The individual health care professionals' narratives of their medical encounters with patients used their interactions, values, and emotions to describe their relations with patients. These narratives were epic narratives (Gabriel, 2000), wherein the professionals played the role of hero in helping the patients. These narratives functioned as strong sensemaking devices for understanding their values in relation to their patients. Health care professionals have strong self-control over patient relations in their daily patient encounters.

The health care professionals' individual ante-narratives regarding interdisciplinary meetings illustrated how the logic of medical professionalism (Reay & Hinings, 2009) was broken down into multiple micro-institutional logics, wherein the different professional groups of doctors, therapists, and nurses spoke of their own professional values being different and involved in ongoing struggles with each other. These ante-narratives illustrated how ambiguity and tensions became part of understanding the meeting and the difficulties health care professionals have of working together in meetings. Meetings became an arena for power games, during which implicit feelings of being a low status group became visible, resulting in silent participants.

These narratives demonstrated how spending time with patients was one of the strongest values of the professional groups and how wasting time with each other perhaps became the weakest value for the professional groups in this study. Together these narratives demonstrated how the value of the patient-professional relationship guided them and allowed them to speak on behalf of patient needs, and also how professional groups and logics became dominating in their interaction with each other.

Combined, the analysis of these individual narratives contributes with an understanding of how making sense of organizational change in everyday organizing contexts is based on fragmentation and multiple sensemaking processes.

A Combined Model of Shared and Individual Narratives

In the analysis of collaborative innovation through design thinking, two shared narratives of participation in local innovation projects were presented. This first two shared narratives of local innovation participation demonstrated how engagement and materialization became important sensemaking elements in mobilizing participants in local innovation projects by relating to the social discourses of self-actualization and concretization (Mantere & Vaara, 2008, p. 347).

Then followed with the presentation of a series of individual ante-narratives of patients and local innovation participants and how both positive and more negative ante-narratives emerged. The patient ante-narratives in the diaries and postcards contained positive and negative elements. The positive narratives were encouraging statements; the negative narratives were disapproving statements that had to be handled with more sensitivity by local managers to avoid mistrust and resistance to patient ante-narratives. The patient ante-narratives were a surprise, as they shared interpretations that differed from those of the health care professionals. But the health care professionals had positive ante-narratives about reading them and expressed a willingness to include them and use them to redirect their sensemaking of patients. The health care professionals had other, more negative ante-narratives toward other aspects of the design, tools and the innovation consultant was disappointed by the way they used the tools. Negative ante-narratives thus also emerged about the value of design thinking.

Combined, the narrative analysis illustrated how shared sensemaking of engagement and materialization created a condition of participation in the two local projects. The ante-narratives of patients from, e.g., the post-cards, made it possible for the health care professionals to redirect their sensemaking and form new understandings of patients. In addition, more negative ante-narratives about design thinking processes also emerged.

Narrative and ante-narrative analyses of individual sensemaking and collective or shared sensemaking have the ability to contribute to an understanding of how local organizational change processes is intertwined with shared sensemaking. In the two collaborative innovation projects, the shared narratives directly influenced the mobilization of participants to participate in the project, but at the same time, individual and more fragmented sensemaking also directed participants together, with reluctance.

Shared Narratives

The analysis of coordination through the creation of health agreements between health service providers in municipalities and regional health care providers (hospitals) resulted in three shared narratives from politicians and administrators.

A shared narrative of secure operations, which involved letting the goals become administrative and creating concrete delivery plans to make sure the agreements are successful, for the press and at the National Board of Health, as they are important surroundings for establishing legitimacy and positive relations.

A shared narrative of equal partnership, where politicians built new trust relations between municipalities and regions, opening the door for pluricentric coordination with many centers of authority.

A shared narrative of control became a way for politicians to handle political maneuvering through installing and controlling meeting agendas. This narrative also took into account that coordination of the health care agreements could be understood as a medical problem not well suited for political statements in the press, as local communities' growth and wellbeing were the main legitimate surroundings for politicians.

Together, these narratives demonstrated how sensemaking was a central aspect of defining coordination in health agreements. The narratives illustrated the condition of how to coordinate through securing operations and installing multiple centers of coordination authority. They also demonstrated how coordination between health care providers became a de-politicalized issue, leaving the responsibility of coordination to the hospital level.

The final analysis of policy expectations toward innovation in society and in health care presented three policy narratives. These were not organizational narratives, as they were not narratives told from the perspective of organizational fields. They were policy narratives, as they were written narratives from the policy field, collected from various policy papers.

The first policy narrative was about knowledge production innovation and found its main inspiration from NPM ideas, where competition was addressed as the main innovation problem. The solution was to innovate new products by supporting new relations between the public research infrastructure and private companies.

The second policy narrative was about partnership innovation, where globalization became a major political concern. The solutions were new partnerships and new collaborative innovation centers, and this policy narrative drew strongly on ideas from NG.

The last policy narrative was about public welfare innovation, redirecting the need for innovation in society to address complex societal problems, and the solution was to forge new relations between users/citizens and welfare organizations to gain new capabilities in innovation.

Combined, the three narratives contribute with knowledge on how policy expectations are also dynamic sensemaking devices that change over time, but even so, dominating narratives can be found. The three policy narratives addressed the conditions of becoming an innovative hospital: by building up a knowledge and research infrastructure (to support private innovation), entering into partnerships with private and voluntary organizations, and fostering the development of innovative employee able to interact with new technology and users to generate new innovative solutions.

The last two analyses contribute with knowledge on how dominating narratives become conditions of organizational change. Dominating policy narratives direct legitimate activities and can be conceived as both drivers of and barriers to local organizational change processes.

In sum, the narrative analyses contribute by illustrating how different local change projects generate many different types of narratives to make sense of change processes. The first studies contribute with knowledge on the relations between individual narratives and shared narratives in an everyday organizing context. The last study contributes with knowledge on the relations between national policy narratives and organizational narratives, stressing that organizational narratives are not isolated narratives; they reflect other types of narratives.

Fragmented Sensemaking Conditions and Dominating Sensemaking Directions

> *What are the sensemaking consequences for organizational change processes?*

The overall narrative contribution to the organizational change literature is that an important organizing condition of change processes is polyphonic and fragmented sensemaking processes, as different stakeholders have different understandings of change processes. Furthermore, narrative analyses also demonstrate the dynamic between stability and change by unfolding all of the narratives, including positive change narratives and more critical counter-narratives, which created meanings of the change intentions and events.

The studies further demonstrated how both fragmented and shared sensemaking became sensemaking conditions in organizational change processes in different ways. First, change processes generated multiple understandings of the good intentions, the hard realities, and the unseen consequences of the change processes. Second, dominating collective and shared sensemaking has the ability to mobilize participation in the change processes, as well as generating some of the legitimate and illegitimate values that the change processes reflected, in defining the problems and solutions of the change process. We make sense through the narrative construction of reality (Bruner, 1991). Table 8.2 illustrates the three narrative analyses used and how each made sense of organizational change.

The table demonstrates how individual narratives allow us to understand the complex and multiple sensemaking conditions of organizational change processes. The combined approach of individual and shared narratives demonstrated how shared narratives can direct sensemaking and participation in organizational change processes—not alone, but as part of individual fragmented sensemaking processes. The last narrative analysis identified shared narratives, demonstrating how collective and shared understandings direct legitimate organizational activities and attention toward certain solutions or values, which can create both possibilities and/or challenges in organizational change processes.

Furthermore, the studies show how both structured and fragmented narratives are found in the material, demonstrating that sensemaking occurs through various kinds of narratives. By including both fragmented and structured narratives, a pragmatic approach allowed us to gain a broader articulation of the many different narratives in the field. The

Table 8.2 Making Sense of Organizational Change Through Narrative Analysis

	Making sense of organizational change
INDIVIDUAL NARRATIVES	Fragmented sensemaking as a condition of understanding the possibilities and value of change
COMBINED APPROACH OF INDIVIDUAL AND SHARED NARRATIVES	Directing sensemaking and participation by shared narratives combined with individual sensemaking; being able to direct participation in organizational change processes
SHARED DOMINATING NARRATIVES	Directing sensemaking in defining legitimate and illegitimate change activities

fragmented narratives were found to express individual concerns and offered a picture of variety and polyphony instead of shared understandings (Belova, King, & Sliwa, 2008; Boje, 2001). The shared narratives were found to express collective concerns, the shared condition, and the shared negotiated values. Shared and fragmented sensemaking are two different ways to explain organizing, and a pragmatic approach that combines them (Bartel & Garud, 2009) makes it possible to address their interaction.

Summing Up and Recommendations for Further Research

To conclude, a narrative approach to organizational change contributes with knowledge of how people construct and share narratives in their work lives in organizations (Czarniawska & Gagliardi, 2003; Czarniawska, 2004; Vaara, Sonenshein, & Boje, 2016). Narratives reflect normal ways of e sensemaking in local contexts, and organizational change happens through the redirection of understandings. Great effort is associated with changing such established sensemaking. This approach is relevant in organizational change processes where change events evoke sensemaking. The narrative analysis can demonstrate how resistance, engagement, participation, and coordination all are activities related to sensemaking as well as the construction of narratives of change ideas and change of routines.

Further studies could build on these snapshots of everyday life in various health care organizations and provide other examples of everyday change processes. They could also contribute by giving us a picture of the living conditions of adapting to and integrating health care technology in an everyday context. An everyday context could also embrace an international comparative health care approach (Ferlie, Montgomery, & Pedersen, 2016). Going back to the beginning, when organizational change becomes a part of everyday life, people regularly negotiate and share narratives to make sense. Changes to the routines of daily operations matter, whether one is a nurse, a physician, clinic manager, a regional administrator, or a patient.

References

Bartel, C. A., & Garud, R. (2009). The role of narratives in sustaining organizational innovation. *Organization Science, 20*(1), 107–117.

Belova, O., King, I., & Sliwa, M. (2008). Introduction: Polyphony and organization studies: Mikhail Bakhtin and beyond. *Organization Studies, 29*(4), 493–500.

Boje, D. M. (2001). *Narrative methods for organizational & communication research*. London: Sage.

Bruner, J. (1991). The narrative construction of reality. *Critical Inquiry, 18*(1), 1–21.

Czarniawska, B. (2004). *Narratives in social science research*. London: Sage.

Czarniawska, B., & Gagliardi, P. (Eds.). (2003). *Narratives we organize by* (Vol. 11). Amsterdam: John Benjamins Publishing.

Ferlie, E., Montgomery, K., & Pedersen, A. R. (Eds.). (2016). *The Oxford handbook of health care management*. Oxford, UK: Oxford University Press.

Gabriel, Y. (2000). *Storytelling in organizations: Facts, fictions, and fantasies*. Oxford, UK: Oxford University Press.

Mantere, S., & Vaara, E. (2008). On the problem of participation in strategy: A critical discursive perspective. *Organization Science, 19*(2), 341–358.

Pedersen, A. R., & Humle, D. M. (Eds.). (2016). *Doing organizational ethnography: A focus on polyphonic ways of organizing*. London: Routledge.

Reay, T., & Hinings, C. R. (2009). Managing the rivalry of competing institutional logics. *Organization Studies, 30*(6), 629–652.

Vaara, E., Sonenshein, S., & Boje, D. (2016). Narratives as sources of stability and change in organizations: Approaches and directions for future research. *Academy of Management Annals, 10*(1), 495–560.

Van de Ven, A. H., Polley, E., Garud, R., & Venkatarman, S. (1999/2008). *The innovation journey*. Oxford, UK: Oxford University Press.

Ybema, S., Yanow, D., Wels, H., & Kamsteeg, F. H. (Eds.). (2009). *Organizational ethnography: Studying the complexity of everyday life*. London: Sage.

Index

Note: Page numbers in **bold** indicate a table on that page.

For Product Safety Concerns and Information please contact our EU
representative GPSR@taylorandfrancis.com
Taylor & Francis Verlag GmbH, Kaufingerstraße 24, 80331 München, Germany

www.ingramcontent.com/pod-product-compliance
Lightning Source LLC
Chambersburg PA
CBHW070732220326
41598CB00024BA/3399